LOST IN PANDEMIC, FOUND IN PANDEMIC

Hope in Times of Tragedy

SRINIVAS MAHANKALI

My sincere dedication to all great souls gracing this world

This book is dedicated to the memory of all the inspiring personalities who have orphaned this world in the midst of the raging Pandemic in the years 2020-2021. Most often, these brave souls like Dr KK Aggarwal, Rajeev Karwal and many Health care workers and Frontline warriors have served the affected selflessly and were always at the forefront of the battle with the Pandemic. They facilitated all those around to face it bravely and many have survived these trying times to take on the challenges in the world in the future. But alas, we have lost these beautiful souls, never to return physically. But, they will continue to stay in our hearts for ever and this is the tribute we can give to them.

This book is also dedicated to the memory of my friends and business associates who have lost their lives and in some cases their loved ones to the pandemic. I share their grief and this book is an effort to preserve their memories.

PREFACE

If there is one period of time, we wish could respond to a rewind and delete button, that is the dreaded period belonging to the years 2020 and 2021, when the world battled the worst ever seen waves of Pandemic starting with Covid-19 and its multiple mutations and resultants.

Starting as unsuspecting cough, the invisible virus turned into a storm inside the bodies of many human beings resulting into the death of millions of them across the world in a matter of under 2 weeks.

During these trying times, we lost a number of valuable lives and many leading lights of the world expired in the most unexpected fashion.

Thousands of frontline workers, health care workers, lawyers, teachers, doctors who were on the frontline, police persons, delivery service providers, industrialists and politicians who were at the forefront of the rescue operations, undertaking yeoman service to the pandemic-stricken citizens across the world expired.

There have been many cases of bravery, charity and commendable service that were demonstrated giving hope to the humanity in depressing times in the face of this dreadful disease.

In this book, we would like to remember and record for ever, those brave and inspiring human beings who always stood out in their lives to light up the lives of all around. It is a duty for us to pay a rich tribute to them, and retain them in our hearts forever, thus showcasing their ever-shining indomitable spirit.

There have also been a number of inspiring actions undertaken by unsung heroes, we would like to recount to the extent possible and draw the inspiration to live with hope and contribute positively to this world, we are a part of.

Lost in Pandemic, Found in Pandemic records the lives of those loved ones we would never forget and the inspiring lessons we learn from several heroic acts from the exemplary citizens & institutions who adorn our world.

If there is one thing, we realise from the experiences during the Pandemic is the ephemeral nature of this life on earth which is not in our control and can end at any moment, however pessimistic it may sound. It is important for us to live in the moment, savoring every moment, learning from others, appreciating others and setting an example for all those around & for the future generation. This will ensure that we remain in the hearts of all those who cared us & those we care as sweet memories, like the wonderful souls we have covered in this book.

"Life is short. Break the rules, forgive quickly, kiss slowly, love truly. Laugh uncontrollably and never regret anything that makes you smile..."- JUVY ANN

ACKNOWLEDGEMENTS

It was in April 2020, that I have written my first book on Covid-19 related topic in the form of a fiction book titled "Corona Wars: Chronicles of a Corporate General". It happened to be one of the world's first STEM (Science Technology Entrepreneurship & Management) fiction books. The book received enormous appreciation with over 35 full ratings on Amazon portal. Many readers of the book requested me to write a sequel to the book as a lot of events that were portrayed in the book were realised or, are mimicking the current real-life scenarios. I wish to sincerely acknowledge and thank all those who read my first fiction book, appreciated it and also are looking forward to more such works from me. It has encouraged me to write further on the subject.

This book has been a result of the anguish and frustration that has been pent up inside me due to the events in the recent past, where a lot of friends and business associates have suffered immensely in the hands of COVID-19 virus and many of them are no more in this world. I wish to acknowledge the impact a number of great personalities, some of whom, I have captured in this book, for their impact on my life. I wish to use the techniques I have researched and presented in this book to overcome the grief and channelise my energies for the greater good of the society.

I wish to thanks my family especially my wife Anuradha, who has been with me through the thick and thin and helped in brainstorming our thoughts to present them in a coherent manner in such a way that, it can also help others like me who are in the process of overcoming their Pandemic induced grief and depression.

I wish to thank Ms. Malathy Singh, who has helped with a lot of research, presentation and coordination and supported me in completing this project. It has been a mammoth and monumental effort. Thank you.

LOST IN PANDEMIC, FOUND IN PANDEMIC

Hope in Times of Tragedy

CONTENTS

My sincere dedication to all great souls gracing this world

PROLOGUE

It was 18ᵗʰ May 2021 and I was grief stricken to read yet another heart-breaking and unexpected news. That of passing away of Padma shri Dr KK Agarwal, the Indian physician and cardiologist who was President of the Confederation of Medical Association of Asia and Oceania (CMAAO), President of the Heart Care Foundation of India and the Past National President of Indian Medical Association.

It has been hardly a week since he urged every doctor in India to undertake the service and treat the patients expeditiously, even if it meant that they have to address multiple patients at a time over the electronic media. ' The Show must go on.' he said, even as he wore his oxygen pipe to supplement his breathing and boost the falling blood oxygen levels.

His death shook the billion odd citizens of the country as he was seen as the messiah who could give the strength to everyone to fight and get rid of this Pandemic.

I remembered the famous song from the Hindi movie 'Three Idiots,' which reminds us of a cheerful personality who lights up the lives of all those around and disappears suddenly without trace.

The key lyrics are recounted below:

Behti hawa sa tha who

Udti patang sa tha woh

Kahan gaya usae dhoondo

Kahan se aaya tha woh

Chhoo ke humare dil ko

Kahan gaya usae dhoondo.

This talks about the person who lived a care free, joyful and lively life filled with compassion for others & touching the hearts of all those around, suddenly disappearing without a trace. The singers urge each other to search and get him back.

While in the movie, it is possible to imagine being able to get back in touch with a person who would have disappeared, in real life it is very unfortunate to recover back those people, who have left our world forever, how much ever we try. Many of the great persons we lost and the millions of those who left their loved ones in this world are like those precious souls, who would never return leaving unforgettable memories.

It was hardly a week, since we lost another indomitable soul to this cruel disease, the news that shook many Indians and made everyone weep. While no one knew that name of this brave soul, a Kashmiri girl, a mother of 30 years, who fought the disease very bravely to only succumb after inspiring everyone around.

It was only a week before her death, that Dr Monica Langeh, who treated her tweeted hopefully on Twitter, "She is just 30 years old & She didn't get ICU bed we managing her in the Covid emergency since last 10days.She is on NIV support, received remdesivir, plasma therapy etc. She is a strong girl with strong will power asked me to play some music & I allowed her. Lesson: 'Never lose the Hope'."

The song she played for the brave young patient, the title song from 'Love You Zindagi', a famous Hindi movie starring Shah Rukh Khan and Alia Bhat, signified the importance of loving every moment of our existence on this mother Earth.

It was heart-rending for every Indian, to lose this brave soul, who signified our life in its true essence and showed us how to fight and never lose hope against adverse circumstances.

Nevertheless, as Dr KK Agarwal messaged to the entire world, 'The show must go on'. We are here in this world to make the most of every moment we live and contribute our level best. This, in face of the humongous tragedy we are facing every day, hearing the news of loss of some associate or the numerous fellow citizens, is indeed a tough ask.

Let us see some of those heroic personalities and heroic acts that can inspire us every moment to live on and fight as long we are here in this world.

CHAPTER 1: DR KK AGGARWAL

"Living for others is worthful life." – Albert Einstein

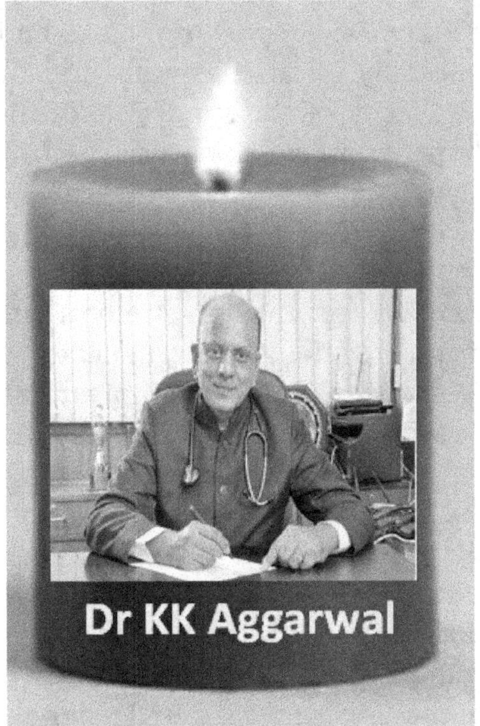

Padma Shree (Late) Dr KK Aggarwal 5.9.1958– 17.5.21

War on Covid-19 Pandemic was led by the eminent Doctors and Health care workers and no one symbolised the medical profession more than Dr KK Aggarwal. If the time could be revered and we could get back one person from the past into life, it would be none other than Padma Shree Dr KK Aggarwal one of the most loved doctors in the whole of India. He served the people & the ill, literally till his last breath. His selfless service and his lively memories will remain with us forever. It is indeed true, when someone said, "An amazing doctor is hard to find and impossible to forgot."

As the past president of Indian Medical Association and as the founding member of the 'Heart Care Foundation of India', Padma Shree Dr KK Aggarwal was always at the forefront of the war on the Pandemic, never resting or taking a long free breath. Many exclaimed with a state of shock after his death with the headline, 'The doctor who always put the patients first till his very end, Dr KK Aggarwal, is no more."

He was an unequivocal supporter of clean and fresh air in the environment, especially in the hospitals and unfortunately, he himself became a victim of the syndrome of infected air in the hospitals that claimed precious lives of over 1000 doctors in the Pandemic as of May 2021.

Dr KK Aggarwal was full of talent. He was Sr. Physician, Cardiologist and Mind Body Consultant and a world class Clinical Echocardiographer, Writer, Author, Anchor, Orator, Columnist, Health Communicator, Social Worker, Educator, Teacher, Trainer, Conceptualizer, Visualizer, Creator, Organizer, Preacher, Administrator, Advisor, Social Activist, Researcher and Meditation teacher par excellence.

He founded multiple organisations & was actively involved in selfless service. He was President of the Confederation of Medical Association of Asia and Oceania (CMAAO), President of the Heart Care Foundation of India and the Past National President of Indian Medical Association. In 2010, the Government of India honored him with the Padma Shri, India's fourth-highest civilian award, for his contributions to the field of medicine.

Taking all precautions for Social Distancing, Dr Agarwal conducted numerous patient consultancies online and gave treatment as well as courage to a number of patients to overcome the disease successfully. He directly or indirectly touched the lives of over 100 million people through his videos and educational programs, offering medical advice and consultancy to alleviate their sufferings from various diseases.

The 62-year-old Dr KK Aggarwal, who was loved by who ever came across him, succumbed after a short stint at AIIMS on Ventilator support. Till a few days before his death, Dr KK Aggarwal demonstrated enormous courage in the face of a deteriorating health condition due to Progressive Covid Pneumonia, that was threatening his life. His passion to serve people and sense of humour that kept up the spirits of his patients and all those who could watch his videos, were infectious and encouraging.

"Observation, Reason, Human Understanding, Courage; these make the physician."— Martin H. Fischer

Dr KK Aggarwal captured the imagination of Indians, captivating them about the potential of impact a doctor can have on the society. Many children across India are inspired by him, to serve the country as doctors, once they grow up.

A statement released by his family after his death reads, "He wanted his life to be celebrated and not mourned. His spirit of spreading positivity in the direst of circumstances must be kept alive in each one of us. Let us remember him for his work and indomitable spirit."

The loss left by the journey of Dr KK Aggarwal to the heavenly abode is impossible to be filled. But the inspiration he has left for all Indians who could ever feel him personally to virtually through his video recordings for times to come is invaluable.

In Sanskrit, there is a saying 'Vaidyo, Narayano, Hari.' It implies that, a Doctor is a form of the supreme God, Lord Vishnu, who is believed to run this world. Dr KK Aggarwal is a true reflection of this belief.

"He is the best physician who is the most ingenious inspirer of hope."— Samuel Taylor Coleridge

A person who always lived for others, Dr KK Aggarwal showed us the path to an ideal life, a life whose purpose is much beyond selfish goals, but the healthy well-being of all those around especially, the poor and the needy. May his soul rest in peace even as he lives in our heart forever.

CHAPTER 2: MR. S.P. BALASUBRAHMANYAM

"The song is ended, but the melody lingers on."- Irving Berlin

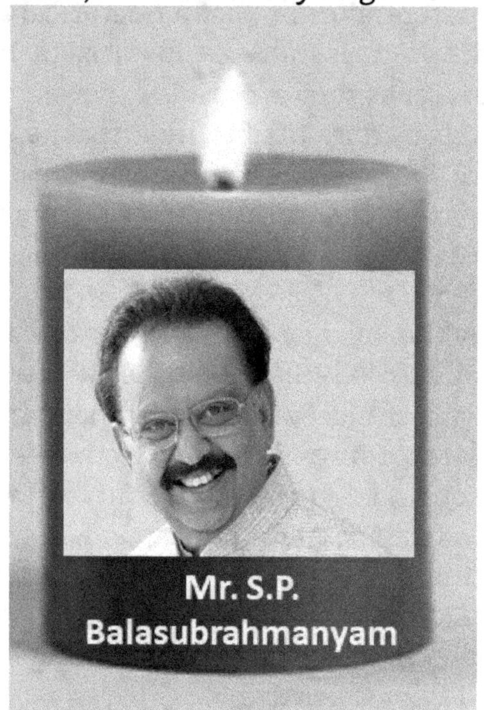

Padma Vibhushan (Late) Mr SPB: 4.6.1946 - 25.9.2020

The Covid-19 virus was at its cruelest when it snatched from this world, one of the most loved and revered entertainers of Indian Cinema, SP Balasubramanyam. SPB or Balu as he was fondly called was always full of life and celebrated not only his excellence in whatever he did, but also guided, mentored and facilitated success of many youngsters.

One of the most humble persons anyone can come across, Balu was always there to support youngsters in cinema or other walks of life. He always took extreme care of his social behaviour. He maintained social distance & highest standards in personal hygiene in all occasions.

A short trip to Hyderabad from Chennai, where he went for a dubbing assignment and one moment of carelessly touching an innocuous audio equipment at the studio was the only known case of his possible encounter with the virus. This could have led to his infection and ultimately to his parting from this world. On 5ᵗʰ August 2020, SPB was tested positive for Covid-19 and was admitted to MGM hospital in Chennai.

Even when he was admitted in a hospital, SPB was cheerful as always, comforting his supporters about his potentially inconsequential hospital stay undertaken as a matter of abundant caution that always defined his personality. As he was admitted to the hospital, he released a 3-minute video on YouTube addressing all his fans, not to worry & he was perfectly fine. This calmed the nerves of millions of people, albeit for a short while.

Things were going on expected lines and he was tested Covid-19 negative on 7ᵗʰ September. However, he continued to be on ventilator support and slipped into critical situation after showing signs of recovery for a brief period. The world was taken aback and slipped into a state of shock when the quintessential entertainer SPB ultimately bid a farewell to everyone around on the 25ᵗʰ of September 2020.

Such is the suddenness of his death that, it was impossible for anyone to even understand how a bubbly and seemingly healthy & joyous human being could suddenly deteriorate and vanish from our midst.

SPB is one of the many finest human beings whose lives have been cut short by Covid19 Pandemic and his loss is indeed unbearable. He holds a Guinness record for the highest number of songs sung by an individual. He sang over 40000 melodious songs we listen across Indian languages like Telugu, Tamil, Kannada, Malayalam, Hindi etc. He touched lives of millions of people with love, fondness and humility. We shall remember forever, that a master entertainer & one of the finest human beings passed through this world. He will remain in our hearts, despite not being there with us physically.

As they say, "When someone you love becomes a memory, the memory becomes a treasure." Memories left by SPB will always remain with us as a treasure in our hearts.

Striving for perfection, passion for the profession, humility, helpful attitude, forever cheerful disposition and an outlook to lighten up the lives of all those around till his very end are some of the great qualities we should emulate, if we want to leave a mark on this earth and be remembered like SPB.

CHAPTER 3: MR. CHETAN CHAUHAN

"Pride makes us artificial and humility makes us real."- Thomas Merton

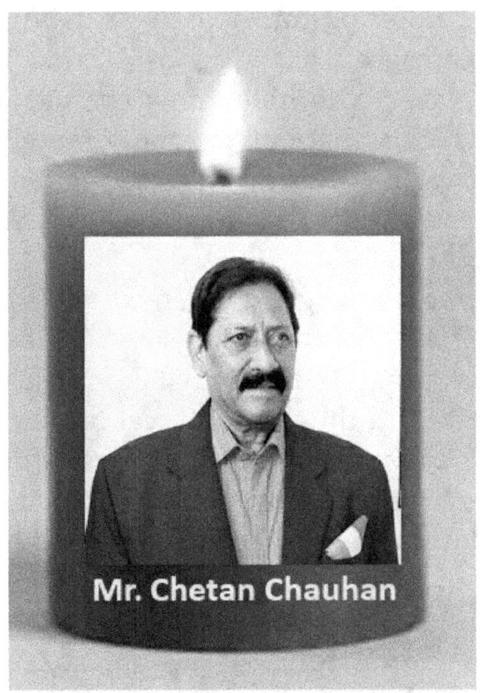

Late Chetan Chauhan- Cricketer & Hon'blw Minister of UP State (21.7.1947 - 16.8.2020)

Covid-19 Pandemic consumed the mightiest and the most loved & Chetan Chauhan sir was one of them. A cricketer who is fondly remembered for his many adventurous innings alongside the Little Master Sunil Gavaskar during the 80's, Chetan Chauhan was one of the most loved cricketers and Indian politicians. He played 40 cricket test matches and along with Sunil Gavaskar earned many accolades for the country on the global cricket scene.

A calm, composed and able administrator, Chauhan sir was

well known for his understated humour and sublime temper. Never to get perturbed in the trickiest of the situations, Chetan Chauhan who has delighted many Indians through his affable nature, served the country as Member of Parliament and the state of Uttar Pradesh as a Member of Legislative Assembly and also as a Minister of the state.

In July 2020, Chauhan tested positive for COVID-19 during the COVID-19 pandemic in India, and a month later he was placed on a ventilator after suffering multiple organ failure. On 16 August 2020, he died in Gurugram at the age of 73.

A great team player, a humble human being, an administrator par excellence, Chetan Chauhan is fondly remembered by many Indians who enjoyed his stoic defense and patience on the cricket field. His passing away left a gaping hole in everyone's hearts that is difficult to fill.

"We come nearest to the great when we are great in humility."- Rabindranath Tagore

"Shri Chetan Chauhan Ji distinguished himself as a wonderful cricketer and later as a diligent political leader He made effective contributions to public service and strengthening the BJP in UP. Anguished by his passing away," lamented Sri Narendra Modi, Hon'ble PM of India, a feeling that reverberates strongly with the hearts of most Indians.

Dedication to the cause taken up, team work, disciplined approach, ability to stand strong against any storm in a calm manner, sense of humor, humility and humble demeanor and a never-say-die spirit are some of the characteristics of great human beings like Chetan Chauhan who will remain in our hearts forever.

CHAPTER 4: MR. RAJEEV SATAV

"Patriotism is supporting your country all the time, and your government when it deserves it."-Mark Twain

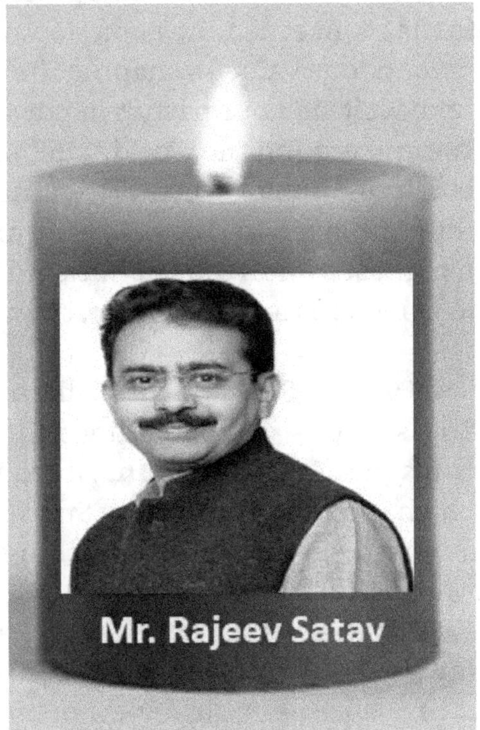

Late Rajeev Satav (21.9.1974- 16.5.2021:
MP Rajya Sabha & IYC leader

Great Politicians and Parliamentarians who devote their lives for the cause of efficient and clean governance of the citizens are a national treasure. Covid-19 pandemic struck cruel blow to the country by snatching many such wonderful assets of India, as it did in many other countries across the world.

A leader from the opposition party in the Parliament, late Sri Rajeev Satav had an impeccable record throughout his career.

"Mankind will never see an end of trouble until lovers of wisdom come to hold political power, or the holders of power become lovers of wisdom."-Plato

Rajeev was a follower of wisdom reflecting the above adage by Plato. He was a member of multiple Parliamentary committees, which are Standing Committee on Railways, Standing Committee on Defence, Committee on Welfare of Other Backward Classes, Joint Parliamentary Committee on Land Acquisition Bill and Consultative Committee on Youth Affairs & Sports. He took active part in any debate that concerned the poor, downtrodden and the farmers adding tremendous value in shaping the final outcomes.

"You don't have to wait till your party's in power to have an impact on life at home and around the world."- Bill Clinton,

Rajeev Satav is a four-time consecutive winner of the Sansad Ratna Award, an honour given to the top-performing Indian MPs. He has the second highest overall tally of initiated Debates, Private Members Bills and Questions among the First time MPs in the Lok Sabha.

As a member of 16th Lok Sabha from Maharashtra, Rajeev attended 81% of the sessions, participating in 205 debates and asked 1075 questions in the 16th Lok Sabha, introduced 23 private member's bills, which include establishing Supreme Court circuit benches in India's metros, compulsory teaching of agricultural education and lowering of age to contest MP, MLA and MLC elections, Granting Paternity Benefit, High Court Bench at Hingoli, Special Package for the State of Maharashtra, Amendment in All India Services Act to ensure periodic review of bureaucrats, drafting of law in plain language bill, Unemployment Allowance Bill, The Agricultural Workers Welfare Fund Bill, 2018 etc.

He was extremely active till April 25, 2021 leading the party's efforts and participating in welfare measures, from the front, till he was diagnosed of Covid-19 and advised rest. Though he tested negative for Covid-19 on 9th May, after treatment, post Covid secondary pneumonia, pulmonary fibrosis and other complications resulted in the loss of life of one of India's favourite voices of the people, soon after, at Jehangir Hospital in Pune.

His death at a young age of 46 came as an unbelievable shock and caused agony to people and leaders irrespective of their party affiliations and it will never be possible to fill the gap caused by his loss.

A dynamic, cheerful, charismatic leader Rajeev had great relations with leaders across the political spectrum. His death was a great loss to Rahul Gandhi to whom he was considered very close.

Rahul Gandhi (Congress leader) tweeted: "I'm very sad at the loss of my friend Rajeev Satav. He was a leader with huge potential who embodied the ideals of the Congress."

India's leaders including Honorable Prime Minister Narendra Modi and top leaders from Congress paid rich tributes to Rajeev Satav. PM Modi tweeted "Anguished by the passing away of my friend from Parliament, Shri Rajeev Satav Ji. He was an upcoming leader with much potential. Condolences to his family, friends and supporters."

"If your actions create a legacy that inspires others to dream more, learn more, do more and become more, then, you are an excellent leader." –Dolly Parton.

Through his urge to work for the welfare of the people till the very end and with impeccable record as a disciplined Parliamentarian, Rajeev made an indelible impact on India's political landscape. His place in the hearts of India's citizens and annals of our history is assured. He inspired many upright citizens to become politicians in the future and many would be inspired by his life to dedicate themselves to the same way.

CHAPTER 5: MS. DEBDATTA RAY

"There is no rank in Sacrifice."- Josephus Daniels

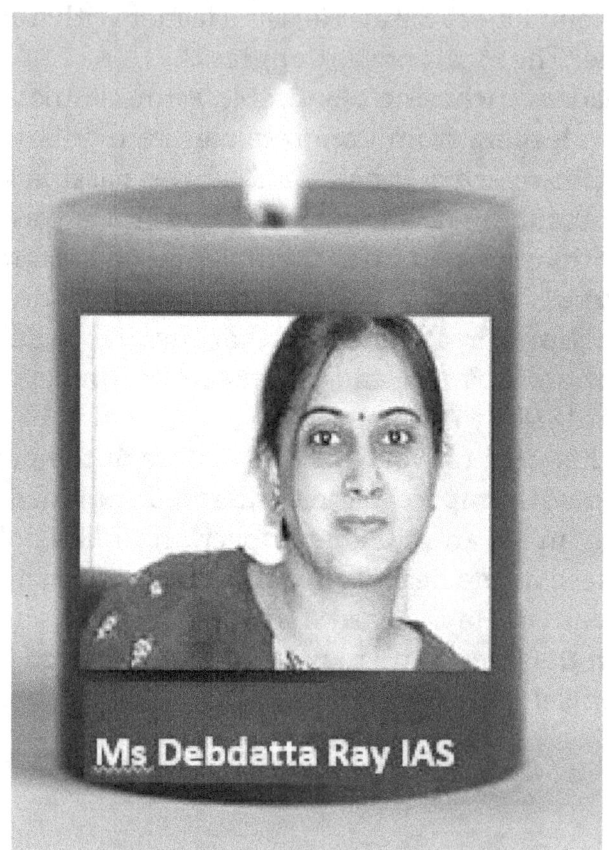

Late Ms Debdatta Ray: Deputy magistrate
at Chandannagore, West Bengal

The Covid-19 pandemic was supposed to be harsher on the males. But it sent shockwaves & devastated many citizens, when a top bureaucrat, a dedicated civil servant who was actively participating in Covid relief work for the poor people and the migrant succumbed to the virus after a quarantined stint at her home in West Bengal. Her conditioned deteriorated suddenly and she was rushed to a hospital in Serampore on 13th July 2020, where she breathed her last.

Just in her mid-thirties and a mother of a four year old son, Ms Debdatta Ray was known to be a very active covid warrior. Plunging herself to support the various activities of the Government in its fight against the Pandemic, Ms Debadatta Ray was taking care of the movement of migrant workers to their home towns due to the widespread lockdowns that were announced to curn the virus spread.

Chief minister Mamata Banerjee of West Bengal, paid rich tributes to the demised brilliant officer.

"Grieved to hear about the untimely passing away of Debdatta Ray, who was posted as Deputy Magistrate & Deputy Collector in Chandannagar. A young WBCS (Exe) Officer, she was at the forefront fighting the pandemic & displayed outstanding devotion in discharge of her duties," Banerjee wrote.

"I, on behalf of the Govt of West Bengal, salute her spirit & the sacrifice she's made in service of the people of Bengal. Spoke to her husband today & extended my deepest condolences. May the departed soul rest in peace & lord give her family strength to endure this loss," the chief minister added.

Debadatta Ray is a shining example of the many civil servants and front line workers who served the covid patients till their last breath, despite knowing fully well that they are risking their lives. They are the real Covid heroes who will forever inspire us with their dedication to duty, selfless service, sacrifice while serving the Government and the citizens.

"Power that doesn't help the people, is not power but pandemic." ― Abhijit Naskar,

CHAPTER 6:DR MANISHA JADHAV

"Sometimes, doctors risk their lives just save others.+- Unknown

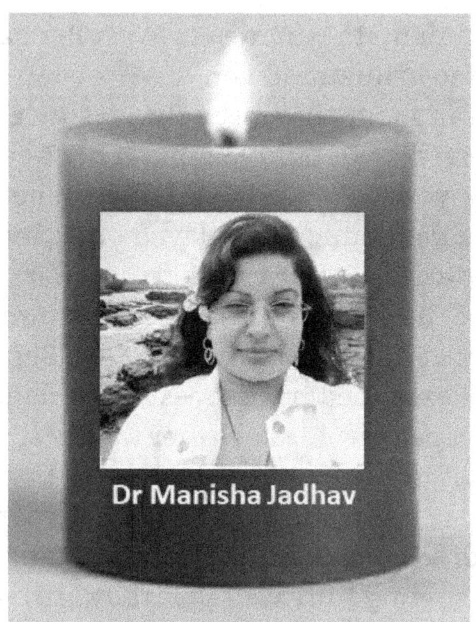

Late Dr Manisha Jadhav (1970 - 19.4.2021)-
CMO, Sewri TB Hospital

India was shocked to learn the death of a leading TB specialist doctor Dr Manisha Jadhav who served the Covid patients till her very end.

On 18th April 2021, 51-year-old Dr Manisha Jadhav, the Chief Medical Officer at Sewri TB Hospital in Mumbai, who contracted Covid-19 shared a post on Facebook that said, 'May be the last Good morning. I may not meet you again in this platform. Take care, all. Body die, but soul does not."

It was on 19th night, the doctor who saved hundreds of lives from dreaded diseases like Tuberculosis, succumbed to Covid as she had predicted.

A trained chest physician and an experienced administrator, Dr Manisha has been at the forefront of handling the pandemic ever since it hit the country in March 2020. She ensured personal protective equipment & all other necessities for the hospital's workers despite heavy shortage. She even took active lead to ensure that patients do not suffer and struggle to reach the hospital, due to the lockdowns that were in place. Despite losing her brother and mother to the Pandemic, she continued to keep her spirits high enough to be able to actively serve the patients and save their lives.

While the helplessness of the medical fraternity against a supposedly manufactured virus that took so many continued to take its toll, the dangerous roles of the doctors and healthcare workers of this country who are working in virally loaded environments became more and more evident.

We must pay a great tribute to doctors like Dr Manisha Jadhav, who epitomes the sacrifice that our frontline workers, especially doctors who are directly exposed to the patients make. They are trying to save thousands of lives of hapless patients, knowing fully well that they are exposed to the direct blast of their viral expulsions, thus inhaling billions of these killer particles that could end their lives.

As Dr Manish Jadhav, put in her social media post, one hopes that her soul indeed returns soon to this world to live a happy life that makes up for the enormous sacrifices that he made in this short and sweet life. Let us pray God to grant our wishes to see again, the countless souls that have left suddenly amidst the Pandemic.

Doctors like Dr Manisha Jadhav and a countless such others, repose our faith in humanity and the healing power of these god's angels and will surely live in our hearts forever, lightening it and inspiring us forever.

CHAPTER 7: MR. RAJEEV KARWAL

"Success is not final, failure is not fatal: it is the courage to continue that counts."-Winston Churchill

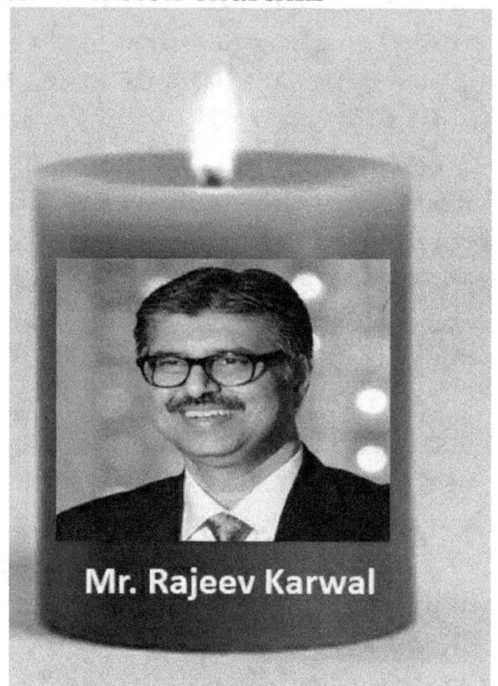

Rajeev Karwal(11.04.1963 - 12.05.2021):
Founder, Milagrow Humantech, India

Entrepreneurs are the greatest gift to any society and are special to their mother country. They provide revenues and employment to many and are net contributors to the society.

Rajeev Karwal always epitomised the spirit of a gutsy entrepreneur, who never gave up against failing odds and in trying times.

Professional Manager par excellence and a successful entrepreneur who overcame many struggles, Rajeev Karwal's career represented an ideal dream to millions of Indian professionals and entrepreneurs.

Having started as a marketing professional with successful

sales & marketing stints in many leading Indian and Multinational organisations like Onida, LG, Philips and Electrolux before starting his venture Milagrow Human Tech in 2009.

He always stuck to ethics and always working on the cutting-edge technologies and aimed to manufacture pathbreaking products at an affordable cost out of India. Rajeev Karwal's venture proved to be on the verge of breaking out into the global map with its fast-growing segments of robots. His robots assisted the hospitals in remaining clean and sterile by spraying disinfectants round the clock in the face of depleted manpower due to the Pandemic.

A 750% growth in a product category of cutting edge technologies like Artificial Intelligence and Machine learning coupled with manufacturing excellence in a year ended March 2021 was the right recipe that a country like India needed the most to catch up with the global leaders.

Milagrow's humanoid robots, iMap 9 and **Humanoid ELF** have been deployed by the **All India Institute of Medical Sciences (AIIMS), New Delhi** to support the hospital staff in disinfection & Sanitization of hospital surroundings and in establishing a communication chanel between the isolated patients and their relatives outside the hospital, respectively.

AIIMS director Dr Randeep Guleria said in April 19th "Milagrow Floor Robot iMap9.0 & Milagrow Humanoid will be tried at AIIMS Hospital, New Delhi,". This facilitated an Indian Made in India Robot to debut in the top most hospital of India and Rajeev Karwar proudly announced to the media, "Milagrow Robots is very happy to support AIIMS in its effort to fight the COVID-19 pandemic and will work closely to develop more products based on the feedback of actual conditions. As the outbreak continues to rise alarmingly, our state-of-the-art robots will help check the virus spread and protect the doctors, nurses and caregivers from getting infected."

Fate took a cruel turn when Rajeev Karwal got infected with the dangerous strain of Covid-19 just after this event and even before his friends and colleagues could realise that he has been bedridden, his condition deteriorated and India lost one of its brightest stars and a darling entrepreneur.

It was heartbreaking for many of his friends and to me who have always been following him closely, admiring him with awe and inspiration for over 25 years, to learn that Rajeev Karwal has left this world for good. It was too sudden to sink in and pushed many Indians and his international associates into a state of shock.

Rajeev Karwal's life teaches us to have a purpose for life and that we should never give up till the very end in striving to achieve the same. He always strived till the very end with the larger goals of achieving excellence even while operating on the most challenging frontiers of human possibility. He leaves everlasting positive impact in this world. This is a life that one can be proud of, as we leave from here world one day or the other.

The legacy and the inspiring life that he led, his fightback against all odds & never-say-die spirit to eventually succeed as an entrepreneur in his life time, makes him a legend. Rajeev Karwal will live in our hearts for-ever, egging us on, inspiring us and motivating us to strive for better world and a great India.

CHAPTER 8: MR. RAMESH NANGARE IPS

"I can assure you, public service is a stimulating, proud and lively enterprise. It is not just a way of life, it is a way to live fully."--- Lee H. Hamilton

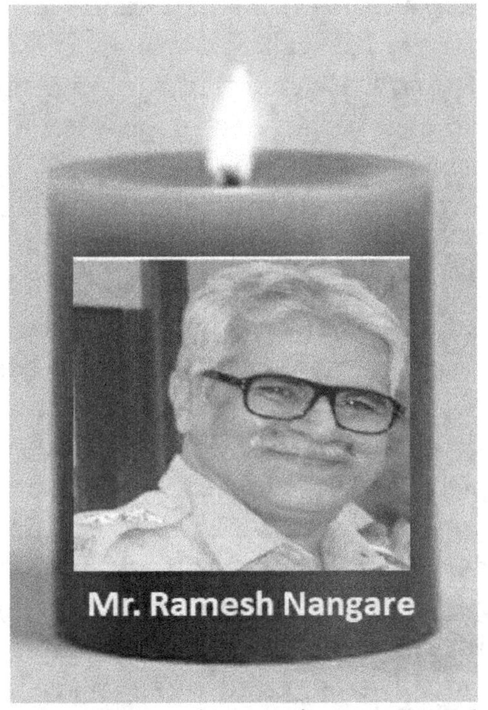

Late IPS, Ramesh Nangare (Age 55): ACP, Mumbai

Law enforcement officers in the state government have a major role in enforcing strict measures aimed at curbing people movement and enforcing lockdown in the peak of the Pandemic. Being directly exposed to public, they also come across the plights of many citizens and this is where we often come across heroes who risk their lives in serving them as well.

Ramesh Nangare, a senior police officer in Mumbai, known for his many heroic deeds during the Covid-19 Pandemic, is one such police officer who will be missed dearly.

An assistant commissioner of police (ACP) in the Sakinaka division, Ramesh was praised for his good work and excellent management for containing the spread of Covid-19 in Dharavi and is known as a dedicated and fearless police officer.

As per Indian Police Service (IPS) officer Niyati Thaker Dave, who was zonal DCP for the Dharavi area at the time, "He has played a pivotal role in strict enforcement of lockdown rules, distribution of masks, sanitisers and food grains to Dharavi residents during the pandemic. He walked through the lanes and raised awareness about Covid. He handled the migrants' issue during the pandemic and also became an inspiration for his colleagues and subordinates. He was featured in NatGeo's documentary for his outstanding work to prevent the spread of coronavirus in the densely populated slum pocket. His death is a huge loss to the police department,"

He died of cardiac arrest, just, two days after he took the second dose of vaccine for Covid-19. Whether his death is due to the after effects of a hidden asymptomatic viral disease that surfaced just after administering the vaccine dose or due to the stress and exhaustion coupled with his ignoring the symptoms of the heart disease while being immersed with delivering his responsibilities, leading to a sudden surfacing of the attack, it will never be known.

But one thing is clear. His selfless work, putting the safety and welfare of the citizens even before his own safety and wellbeing, will forever be remembered, granting his place in our hearts forever.

He also epitomises the spirit of the Police, who in recent times, fought like hell with the invisible virus from the front, by risking their lives and continue to deliver yeomen service to this country.

"To ease another's heartache is to forget one's own."— Abraham Lincoln

CHAPTER 9: DHARAVI'S RAVINDRA

A Typical Covid Martyr
"A hero is someone who has given up his life for something bigger than oneself."- Joseph Campbell

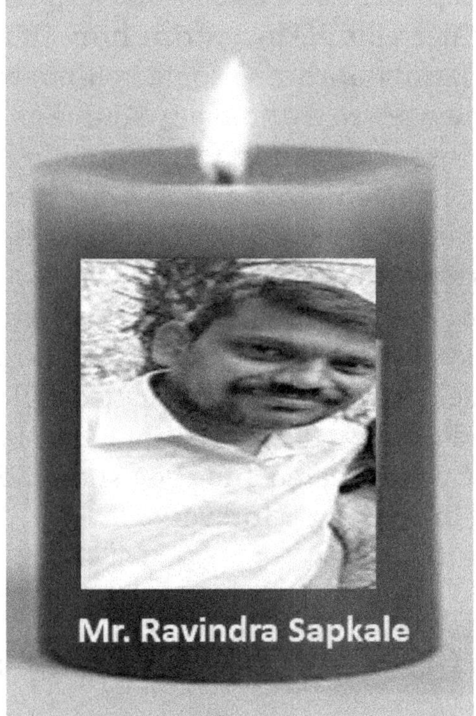

Late Ravindra Sapkale (45); Covid Heo, Dharavi, Mumbai

Ravindra Sapkale was a 45 year old resident of Dharavi, Mumbai's largest slum that was severely affected during the first wave of the Covid-19 pandemic. An employee of a cable company, he lived a happy life with his wife Yogita and children Pranay and Pranali Sapkale.

Seeing the plight of the sufferers in the slum during the lockdown, Ravindra and his friends took it upon himself to serve the needy, who are going hungry due to the non-availability of ration material and also because of their inability to earn due to joblessness.

He went out every day despite the request from his family members to stay safe inside their house, to serve the call of the needy who would otherwise go hungry. They served them food and ensured no one in the colony goes hungry due to the prevailing situation, till the dreaded disease struck him in the first week of May 2020. Soon he had to be hospitalised and died after 45 days in the hospital despite the best efforts of the doctors.

Ravindra sacrificed his life by putting himself in the line of fire, leaving a proud family of three people behind, but who are now left to fend for themselves without any source of earnings.

There are many such unsung warriors who left behind their orphaned families and children and it is the need of the hour to put in place a system to take care of them in the future and ensure that the families are not left in desperate waters.

Government of India and many state governments have put in place processes, systems and schemes to take care of women widowed in the Pandemic and also the orphaned children.

Sacrifices made many covid warriors like Ravindra Sapkale should always be remembered and they should be celebrated for ever with a place in our hearts forever.

CHAPTER 10: MR. VIVEKANANDAN

"We all die. The goal isn't to live forever, the goal is to create something that will."- Chuck Palahniuk

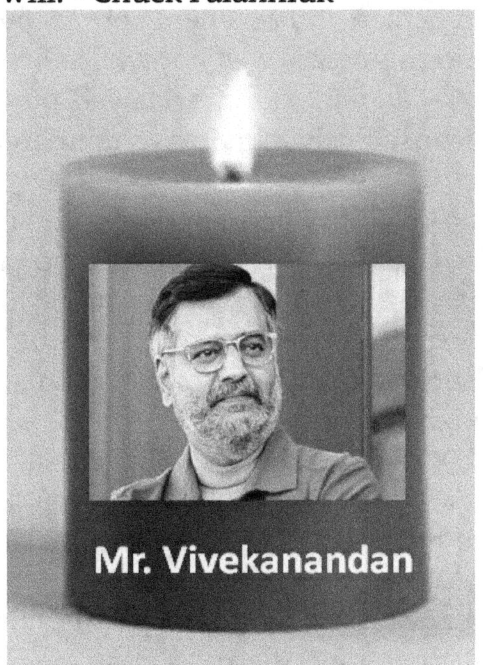

Padma Shri Vivekanandan (19 November 1961 – 17 April 2021),: Versatile Tamil Actor

Covid-19 pandemic struck without any partiality across all the Indian states, taking away chosen personalities who endeared themselves to the public, capturing their imagination through their inspiring deeds. Strange have been its ways of infecting people that, most often one does not know the real cause of death or if at all, there is a connection to Covid-19, when they die in the Pandemic times. Vivek, a popular Television and Cinema artist, well known for his social service contribution left for God's abode on 17ᵗʰ April 2021, due to a massive heart-attack, just a day after taking the Covid-19 preventive vaccine shot. His shocked friends and fans attributed an indirect Covid-19 connection to his death.

Vivekanandan popularly known as Vivek was an Indian film actor, comedian, television personality, playback singer and social activist working in the Tamil film industry.

An environmentally conscious and socially minded person, Vivek founded the Green Kalam initiative in 2010 with the mission of planting one billion trees across Tamil Nadu.

A quick-witted person and excellent communicator with a terrific sense of humour, Vivek is well known for hosting popular TV Shown in Tamil Television. He interviewed movie personalities and was always consciously striving to contribute positively to the society.

Tragedy struck Vivek in 2015 when his teenage son Prasanna Kumar died at the age of 13 due to Dengue and Brain fever. Overcoming the unbearable loss, Vivek slowly pulled himself out of the depression and despair to once again plunge himself actively into working for the society and also in contributing to the entertainment world through a variety of roles.

On 16th April 2021, Vivek took his Covishield vaccine shot and urged all his followers and the public in general to follow suit and shrug off vaccine hesitancy to protect themselves by taking the shot.

It is indeed a strange & sad coincidence that Vivek who seemed perfectly fine till then, died the following day due to a massive heart attack. Though the jury was immediately put out clearing the role of vaccine in causing his heart-attack, doubts continue to linger in the minds of his fans about the connection between the two events.

Filmmaker Shankar Shanmugham captured the grief of Vivek's innumerable fans & followers when he tweeted, "Today we lost an amazing actor, wonderful human being and lover of nature: Padma Shri Vivek. His contributions to my films, Tamil Film Industry and to society is immeasurable, so is this loss. May his soul Rest In Peace. My heartfelt condolences to his family, friends and fans."

Strange are the ways of God that venerated human beings undertaking excellent work with social consciousness for the public good, leave our world at a relatively young age, leaving behind them, a vacuum in the hearts of the people.

Dr Vivek who was awarded Padma Shri for his contribution to the society and the entertainment world will forever live in our hearts and continue to inspire us to add value to all those around through our thoughts, words & good deeds.

CHAPTER 11: IBRAHIM BADUSHA

"You only live once, but if you do it right, once is enough." — Mae West

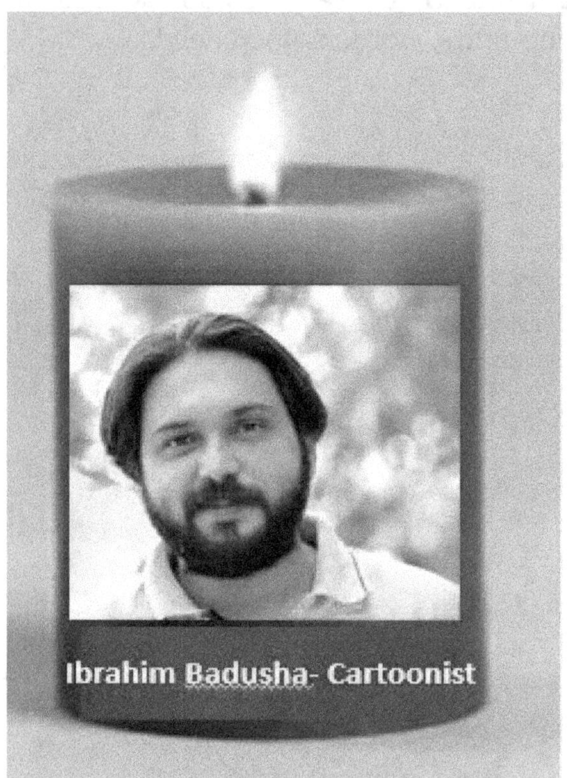

Late Ibrahim Badusha (37): Cartoonist, Kerala

For many months during the Covid-19 pandemic, Ibrahim Badusha, one of the most well-known cartoonists of Kerala state was using his skill to spread awareness about Covid-19 through his amazing cartoons. Many lives would have been saved due to the precautions that people have taken thanks to the awareness. However, the cruel fate consumed one of the most loved persons in the God's own country in the form of post Covid-19 infection complications.

He lived to spread joy in the hearts of people through his cartoons for Children through alphabet cartoons, for public through political cartoons and also through his support for charitable activities.

Ibrahim Badusha was instrumental in founding Kerala Cartoon Club and also served as Vice chairman of the Kerala Cartoon Academy. When Kerala was hit with disastrous flood in June 2019, Badusha travelled extensively to raise funds to support the Chief Minister' Disaster Relief Fund through the cartoon club along with the fellow cartoonists in the state.

His death owing to post Covid pneumonia, shortly after recovering from Covid-19 plunged his numerous fans into a state of shock. A person who was passionate about his cartoons and spread joy to everyone around through his art, Badusha will remain etched in the hearts of his followers, many of them children across the globe.

CHAPTER 12: MR. NAVEEN T.

"It shakes us apart to see someone who has been a huge part of our life disappear in a second."

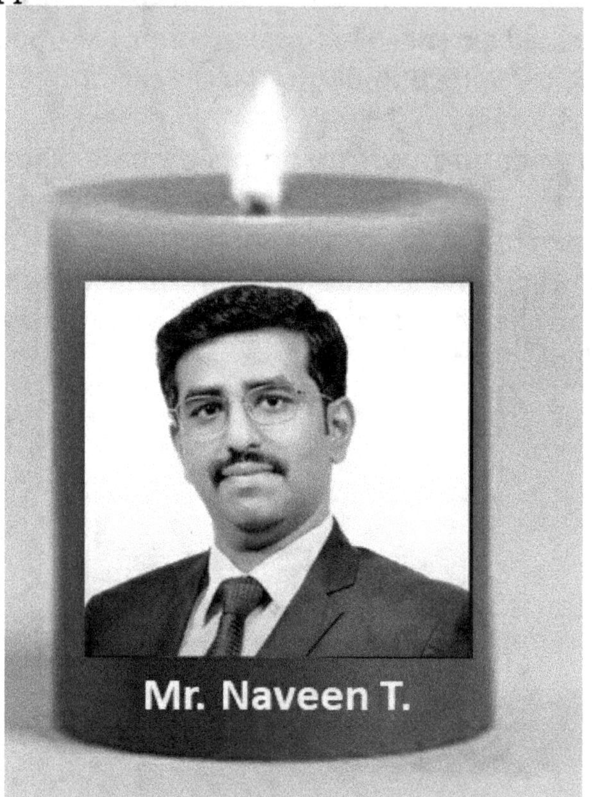

Late Naveen T (35): My ex-colleague at ULTS

Covid-19 Pandemic struck vicious blows to many lives destroying many people, families, friend and relationships.

Naveen all of 35 years old, was my amazing colleague at ULTS (Belonging to ULCCS group, one of the greatest co-operatives from India , a close to 100 year organisation from Kerala State).

Brilliant, cheerful, health conscious, friendly, helpful and forever smiling Naveen spread joy and confidence wherever he went. An expert in IOT, Networking technologies and business development Naveen was a great & dependable colleague and an excellent team player.

When I shifted to Bengaluru to join NISG an organisation owned by Government of India and NASSCOM, Naveen was nice enough to visit me in office during his visits to Bengaluru, even during the Pandemic when the lockdowns were barely released. Extending his helpful hand and being there for me as he does to his friends and family, Naveen was one of those who not only read the books I authored, but also vented out his nice feelings about them in the form of reviews on Amazon.

Family considerations and the need to take care of the elder family members during the Pandemic forced him to find a job and move to Bangalore.

Naveen barely became a father during the second half of March 2021, when he and his elder family members were diagnosed with Covid-19 and had to be hospitalized in an ICU during early April 2021.

The death of his in-laws and other patients in front of his eyes in the ICU one after the other shook the spirits of Naveen. shattering his morale and dented his willingness to fight the virus. It was otherwise common for many people of his age and fitness, to recover from the viral infection. However, the motivation was not enough for him to shake up the losses of his loved ones in front of his eyes. On April 7th, Naveen who was seemingly recovering from the infection, suddenly collapsed due to a sudden drop in Oxygen levels and a heart attack. The second wave of Pandemic saw many such incidences when seemingly recovering patients collapsed suddenly to death. Film editor Ajay Sharma too expired in the same way on 5th of May 2021 at an hospital in Delhi.

This was an unbelievable news for many of his colleagues, family members and dear friends who will take ages to shrug off this loss. A person with whom you have been working, sharing notes and moving around, vanished suddenly from their lives after a short trip the hospital.

This has been one of the common scenarios during the Pandemic in India. Despite maintaining healthy lifestyle, fitness and taking all precautions like staying at home most of the time, people got infected by the virus which was floating in the air. Once infected, the reaction of the body & the response to ward it off has been so erratic and unpredictable, that a lot of lives have been lost all of a sudden in an inexplicable manner.

It is truly a life shattering experience for many across the world to lose friends like Naveen all of a sudden. To see his wife, just become a mother only to lose her parents and husband even before she could step out of the bed after her child's delivers is even more disheartening and depressing to think of.

Naveen always loved and lived his life as a sport, gliding through his stint on the earth in a cheerful manner, giving fond memories to his friends & family. He will always be remembered by those he touched. His life is an inspiration for everyone to live to the fullest and be a responsible & living human being.

Our hearts will ache forever and tears flow when we recount your memories. Rest in Peace Naveen. You will remain in our hearts forever. Your way of life is an inspiration for us to live on celebrate the rest of our lives.

CHAPTER 13: MR. MUNISH SAXENA

"One day we were having animated discussions amidst colleagues and business associates and the next day he was gone for ever."- Poignant stories from the Pandemic times.

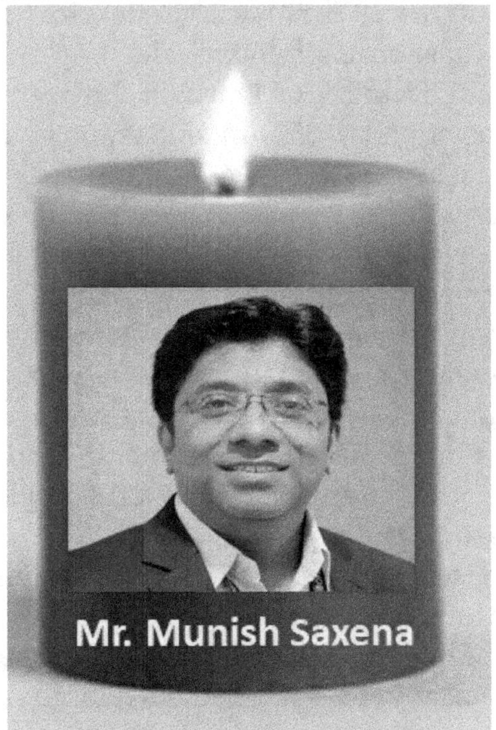

Late Sri Munish Saxena- Global Sales Head
(PSI-Pratham Software, Jaipur)

Covid-19 dealt shocking blows to many friends, families and colleagues of several senior persons & CXOs across Indian industry.

Munish Saxena was one of close friends who lost their lives and sometimes sacrificed, we can say as they caught infection while serving the infected patients to ensure that they got proper treatment.

It was in early April that I and my team were engaged with PSI, Jaipur, their promoters and CXOs to explore business opportunities in emerging technology landscape together. Even as were in the midst of the discussions, we could see Munish reduce his participation in the meetings to participate in the covid relief activities in the city, become weak a bit and excuse himself for a few days to get back his health once again to get going.

It was not be and it was shocking for us to suddenly realise that he passed away on the 19th of May 2021 despite the best efforts of the doctors in a super specialty hospital.

The post by the founder of Pratham Software (PSI), captures the wonderful personality of Munish Saxena, which is also a reflection of the feeling of many colleagues, business associates across the world.

"Munish you will always remain as fond memories with PSI. You are the strongest pillar and a great asset of Pratham Software and we can't imagine a single day in office without you. You are a synonym of loyalty and trust. We have won so many project deals with you in last 19 years but no idea how we lost you in last battle of 19 days in hospital with Corona. We did everything but we couldn't save you."- Sumeeti Mittal, Co-Founder & Director at Pratham Software (PSI).

This is not an isolated case and has been a common occurrence across organisations where we lost senior persons in the organisation who were leading from the front to deliver their official, charitable and personal activities with equal aplomb,

As Ms Sumeeti captured beautifully in her message that day, "I wish, there is a rewind button and we do something extra and bring Munish back."

This is a common feeling for many Indians who lost their loved ones. It is indeed a sad, well known and definitive fact that we on earth have not been able to discover a rewind button in real life and life will not give one more chance. We feel helpless to realise how an invisible particle can end our lives abruptly when it joins forces with the fate. All we can do is to be inspired by great souls, live in the present, lead lives without harming anyone else, but helping others, thus inspiring all those around.

Munish Saxena will be remembered by many for this very way of life he lived and as tears roll down our cheeks, we realise that he will always remain with us in our hearts.

CHAPTER 14: SV PRASAD IAS

"If I'm going to be a leader then I have to go places that other people are afraid to go to. That's what makes a leader. To be not afraid to step out and go over the frontline. To stare darkness right in the face." -R. Kelly

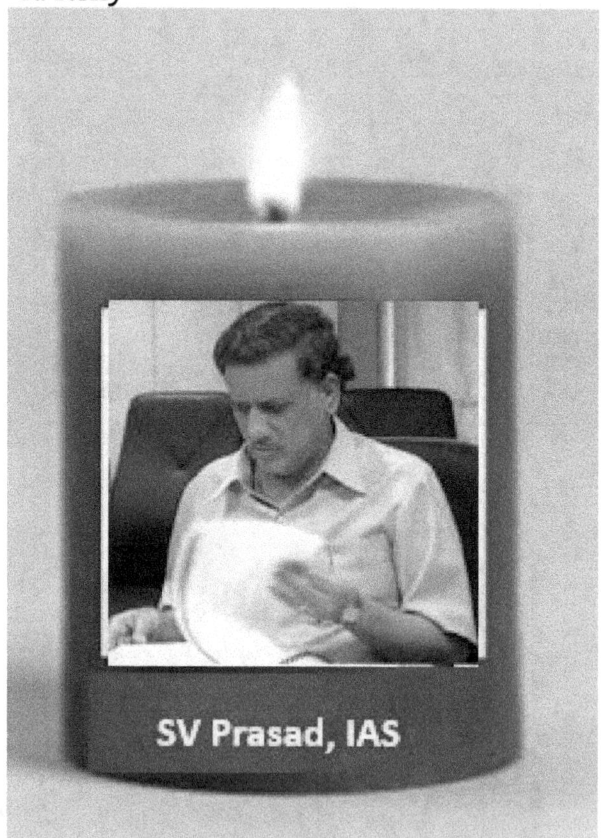

Late SV Prasad IAS- Vigilance Commissioner of AP

Covid-19 has not differentiated between rich or poor, ordinary citizens or IAS, elder or young and sometimes vaccinated or not.

Arun Kumar Singh IAS, the acting Chief Secretary of Bihar state, SV Prasad, Retired Chief Secretary of Andhra Pradesh & Acting Vigilance Commissioner of AP state are some of the eminent

& well acclaimed civil servants, who lost their lives to this dreaded virus during the Pandemic.

SV Prasad, a 1975 batch IAS officer was considered one of the most accomplished civil servants India ever saw. Having served as Chief Secretary under three Chief Ministers of undivided Andhra Pradesh with aplomb, SV Prasad sir enjoyed a dream career for any civil servant of India.

Though he was vaccinated twice, he contracted the dreaded virus three times and proved unlucky the third time. He along with his wife, a highly acclaimed person in the IAS circles as an able leader of IAS officer Wives' association succumbed to Covid-19 with a gap of less than a day on June 1st 2021, a day that can be termed as the most forgettable day for many fans of professionalism in Governance.

Well known as an outstanding public servant, an extraordinary professional in the Government, impactful and charismatic presence, strong character, SV Prasad sir was well liked for his disarming nature and was referred to as Ajatha Shatru or a person without any enemies. His time tested and proven credentials, consistent performance, and balance in tricky situations, enabled him to endear himself to serve his political bosses even though they differed in their temperament substantially.

To recognise his brilliance as a person of highest levels of integrity and also to have his continued guidance even after his retirement as Chief Secretary of the State, the Government appointed him as the AP State government's Vigilance commissioner.

The death of Mr & Mrs SV Prasad IAS on the 1st of June 2021 due to the Covid-19 is a deafening blow to the entire IAS and Civil Services fraternity. It also reflects the high levels of risk the public servants who often lead from the front or are people oriented, face.

Another key factor highlighted is the fact the vaccination is no panacea and even those who are infected once and are known to possess antibodies against the virus. High levels of viral presence in the atmosphere, repeated mutations of the virus and the resemblance to common cold that makes vaccines ineffective at times pose renewed challenges to those creating vaccines against this dreaded disease.

Wonderful human beings like SV Prasad sir who was always cheerful, humble, apolitical, efficient, friendly, dynamic and professional are a treasure for any country. The country will surely miss such gems of human beings and we will forever continue to cherish their memories. He will continue forever in the hearts of all those who interacted with serve as a role model for numerous civil servants on whose shoulders the administration of the country runs.

CHAPTER 15: MR. IBRAHIM RAHUMATHULLAH

How much pain have cost us the evils which have never happened."—Thomas Jefferson

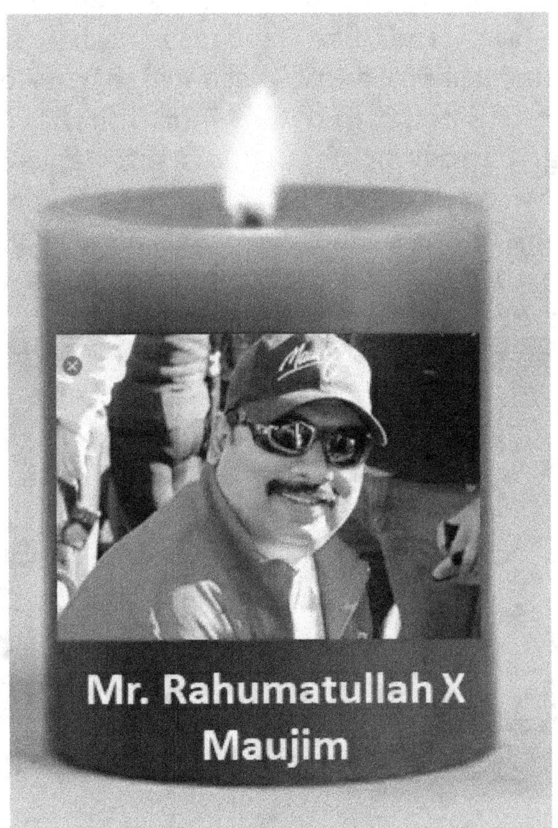

Ibrahim Rahumathullah (Dec 1967 - April 2021) : Entrepreneur & Ex Maujim Head

Covid-19 virus infected crores of people affected their health, resulting in the death of many patients.

But, there were also cases where the death could not be directly attributed to the infection or the disease. Death of friends like Rahumathullah during the Pandemic times came as a shock to me and my friends and it is yet to sink into our minds. It also makes us delve into the various hidden causes that plagued the citizens, many of which may not seem to be linked to the viral infection in any way. The sudden death of friends like Rahumathullah without any prior signals or known co-morbidities brings the focus onto a number of other associated silent killers.

Ibrahim Rahumatullah fondly known as IR, was a dynamic corporate executive who was behind the success of leading global fashion accessory brands like RayBan, Bausch & Lomb eye care and Maujim Sun glasses. He always seemed to be living the proverb by Alan Watts, "It's better to have a short life that is full of what you like doing, than a long life spent in a miserable way."

He was known to be a jolly and fun-loving person, much liked by his colleagues and customers alike. His happy go lucky attitude and friendly nature also endeared him to the most sought aft personalities in the film and sports domains.

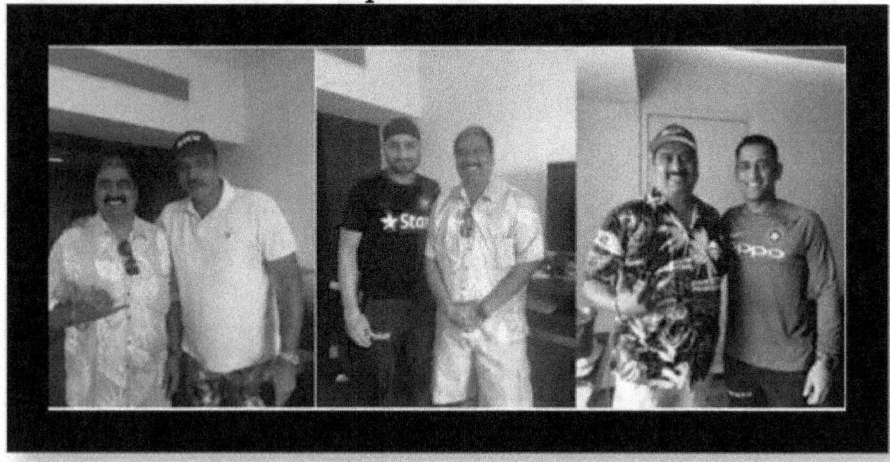

Always smiling, friendly and humble

Deciding to become an entrepreneur, IR quit his job and invested his money heavily into fashion retail and things seems to going well as the business started booming and it is then the Pandemic raised its ugly head leading to the era of lockdowns and death of brick-and-mortar focused retail businesses.

With lockdowns becoming a way of life and got extended indefinitely, small startups were adversely affected due to heavy fixed expenses and a lot of staff to be taken care of. Their promoters became more and more difficult and stressful.

Stress is often the silent and the biggest killer of the mankind. Though the people under heavy stress ay at most times, camouflage their feelings, it builds up underneath the skin, destroying the vital parameters of the body and its immunity as well. One fine day, IR who was working late into the night on his official work, slipped silently into the arms of death and the reason that was later pronounced to be the cause of his death was a massive heart attack.

The sudden death of a dear friend threw many of his friends like the author into a depression for days to come and it is indeed difficult for the jolly memories of togetherness to fade into the oblivion.

Apart from the danger of the contagious virus, we also need to be aware of the damage to the mental health, the Pandemic could inflict upon the citizens indirectly. Deaths arising out of such depressing events and incidences could never have been counted and linked to the Pandemic. But they would indeed be a sizeable number warranting a focused action by the Government and the society.

Another important factor, the death of a dear friend like IR got us to notice closely is the importance of preparing and recording Wills and testaments by everyone to ensure a smooth transition of assets to the dependents and the survivors in the family. Most of the times, the absence of a recorded Will puts the surviving family members in a compromised position and a severe disadvantage as there will not be much clarity regarding the amount of finances left back by the departed soul, as also his or her intention to distribute the same. Though it looks like a depressing and negative thought, it is imperative for all of us to plan for a lawyer mediated and well recorded will, just like how we plan for our insurance.

My every visit to Chennai, Rahumathulla's city of residence was never complete without catching up with IR. We will surely be missing him for ever. May his soul Rest in Peace and hope he comes back soon!

CHAPTER 16: GREAT MEDIA MEN WE LOST

"Journalism will kill you, but it will keep you alive while you're at it." — Horace Greeley

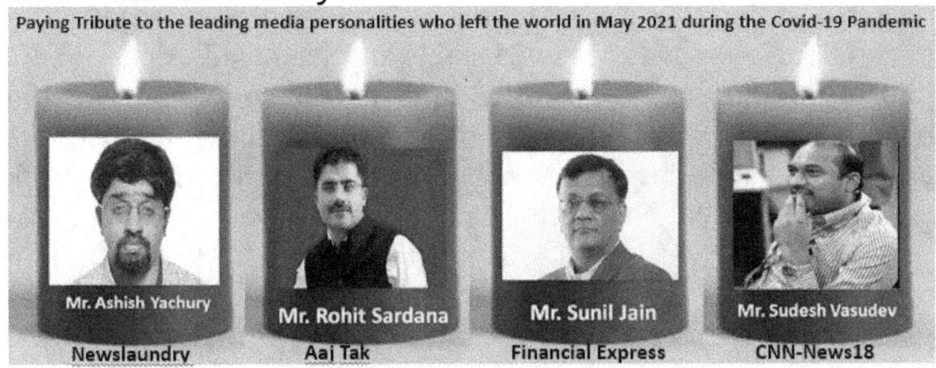

Mediamen and Journalists who laid down their lives

Covid-19 has always been harsh on the frontline workers who are out on the streets covering the stories as they unfold, write them, edit them and present in a palatable manner to the public.

There have been many instances where journalists and the associated media vehicles like the newspapers, radio channels and the TV channels have worked hard to highlight the plight of hapless patients and brought about the intervention from authorities to ensure right action is taken on the frontlines to save lives.

Journalists are most often passionate about their profession and are communicators past excellence. They are always curious about the happenings around the world and love to expose them to public at large.

"I became a journalist to come as close as possible to the heart of the world." — Henry Luce

But this often puts them at close contact with people directly and in crowded places and this is detrimental to their lives during a contagious pandemic like nCovid-19.

It is with a heavy heart that we recount the loss of lives of passionate media persons like Ashish Yechury, Rohit Sardana, Sunil Jain, Sudesh Vasudev and many more wonderful persons who touched the hearts of the citizens by following their passions.

Their friends, associates and viewers fondly recount their passion for the profession, brilliance at work, gentleness and humaneness towards their colleagues.

Ashish Yechury, alumnus of Asian College of Journalism, Chennai, is described by his friends as a mild-mannered and warm professional who was knowledgeable and well read. A passionate journalist and the son of a leading politician in India, could have chosen any profession or position in a leading organisation. Passionate about journalism and wanting to make his own mark in this world, Ashish shunned public attention and materialistic comforts to work as a journalist at new laundry, an Indian media watchdog that provides media critique, reportage and satirical commentary. His friends and colleagues fondly recount the affable nature of Mr Ashish Yechury and his brilliance at work and it took a long time for them to digest the loss of their colleague on April 22, 2021, during the second wave of the Pandemic.

The month of April did not end before it saw the death another brightest star of India's media industry, Rohit Sardana who died of heart attack while undergoing Covid-19 treatment on 30th of April. Rohit Sardana worked at Aaj Tak and ZeeTV. He received Ganesh Vidyarthi Puraskar Award in 2018 which is an annual journalism award conferred by the President of India. His death sent the entire political and media fraternity into a state of disbelief and shock. President Ram Nath Kovind, PM Narendra Modi, Delhi's Deputy Chief Minister Manish Sisodia, Rajasthan's Chief Minister Ashok Gehlot, Ministry of Youth Affairs and Sports Kiren Rijiju, Union Home Minister Amit Shah, Defense Minister Rajnath Singh among many expressed their condolences on his death. Sun has set on the life of another brightest Indian journalist, thanks to the demon Covid-19 that continues to consume many more frontline workers as we speak.

58-year-old Sunil Jain, Managing editor of Financial Express is one of the top newsprint persons whose life has been cut short during the Pandemic on 15ᵗʰ May 2021. He was India's leading financial journalist focusing on regulation, state policy interventions and industries including oil and gas, power, and telecommunications.

Recounting his death and fond memories, Dr Muneer Mohammed, well-known columnist and management consultant. lamented that he lost one of his finest friends who always encouraged him to write thought provoking articles on the subjects of Marketing, Business Management and Economics. His loss leaves a gap that cannot be filled in the top echelons of the business media and his contributions and comradery with the intelligential will be cherished forever.

Closely following the death of Sunil Jain sir, India lost another of its favorite media persons, Sudesh Vasudev, Head Video editing and the founding team member of India's leading news channel, CNN-News18 on 16ᵗʰ May due to complications during Covid-19 treatment.

Fondly remembered by his colleagues and friends at CNN-News18 as an affable, charming & helpful person who mentored many professionals during their career, Sudesh leaves many people in this world heart broken and in despair. News18 media tweeted, "He had a heartwarming smile on his lips in all situations, he also fought Covid with a smile but passed away due to Covid related complications. CNN-News18 grieves the loss of Sudesh Vasudev."

India lost many leading journalists, doctors, lawyers, nurses, Healthcare workers, politicians, bureaucrats and social workers during the 2 years of the Pandemic and is still counting its losses.

The loss is irreplaceable and the feeling depressing. Though it is difficult for all of us to recover from these shocks, it is important for us to stay strong and learn from the way these great men and women have conducted in their lives. The passion with which they worked till the last day of their lives to communicate and help the citizens and businesses is commendable and deserves a strong tribute.

"Journalism can never be silent: that is its greatest virtue and its greatest fault. It must speak, and speak immediately, while the echoes of wonder, the claims of triumph and the signs of horror are still in the air."- Henry Grunwald.

CHAPTER SEVENTEEN

Mr. Bikramjeet Kanwarpal

"I would rather die of passion than of boredom." – Vincent Van Gogh

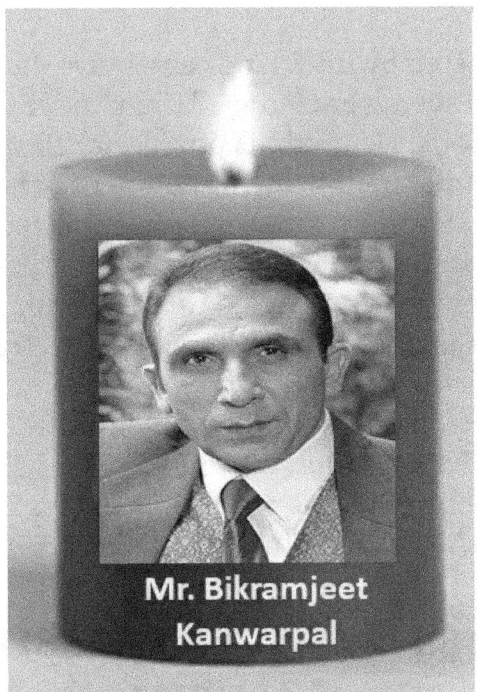

Late Major Bikramjeet (29.8.68 - 30.4.2021):
Retd. Army oficer & Film celebrity

Major Bikramjeet fought and won in the Kargil war for India. On his retirement from the army, he chose to follow his passion for acting. He became a consummate and critically acclaimed actor in a short time, acting in many movies before the world lost yet another impeccable gentleman to the dreaded Pandemic on 30th April, the day that saw the death of other leading lights of the media like Rohit Sardana.

Born in Solan, Himachal Pradesh, India as the son of an Indian Army officer, Kirti Chakra winner, Lt Col Dwarka Nath Kanwarpal, was commissioned into the Indian Army in 1989 and served the country till 2002 as a Major. Acting in films had always been his dream and he started his Bollywood stint in 2003. He acted in a number of films such as Corporate, Page 3, Aarakshan, Jab Tak Hai Jaan, Rocket Singh: Salesman of the Year, Murder 2, 2 States and The Ghazi Attack & also starred on television, in shows such as Diya Aur Baati Hum, Yeh Hai Chahatein, Dil Hi Toh Hai and Anil Kapoor's 24.

He is remembered by his friends as a brave, fantastic and energetic person who always encouraged them to achieve their goals & chase their passions. He used his popularity to spread the awareness about social distancing during Covid-19 pandemic and urged everyone to stay at home to prevent being infected by this dreaded virus, while helping the country to control its spread.

His intense persona as depicted in the movies he acted and his inspirational life journey in the two most impactful professions as a soldier and as an actor leaves behind a lot of memories that not only are captures on celluloid forever, but also inspire others to follow their passions till their life's end.

"Passion is energy. Feel the power that comes from focusing on what excites you." – Oprah Winfrey

CHAPTER 18: Mr. T. Narasimha Reddy (TNR)

"I think a hero is really any person intent on making this a better place for all people." – Maya Angelou.

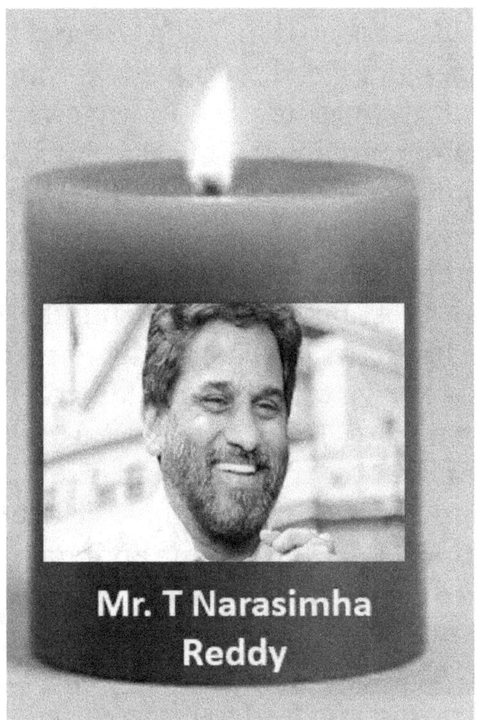

TNR (1.9.1976- 10.5.2021)- Telugu interview
host, film journalist and actor

Covid-19 pandemic came down heavily on the Telugu film industry, when it snatched away one of its famous personalities, TNR aka Thummala Narsimha Reddy, who interviewed many of the leading light of the industry through his YouTube aired online program "Frankly Speaking with TNR".

Passionate about pursuing a career in the film industry, TNR worked as a journalist for many Telugu television channels. He was popular for his creative crime show Neralu Ghoralu in ETV and crime-stories in NTV.

His interview show with the leading Telugu actors was very popular both among the film personalities and with the audience, garnering millions of views. TNR also acted in character roles in many popular Telugu movies and was critically acclaimed for his role.

"Interviewing someone is a very proactive process and requires taking a lot of agency into your own hands to get past people's general normal self-preservation mode."- Brandon Stanton

His ability to get along well with people was amazing and he was well known for stretching the interviews with his participants, mostly well-known busy film celebrities, into hours. Many of them have done their longest media interviews with TNR in which they shared interesting content that further popularised his programs and endeared him to people.

Having taken utmost precautions during the Pandemic, a one of visit to his relatives, who was later diagnosed with Covid-19 infection seemed to have triggered his infection and this put all his fans in a dizzy state. He comforted the people through his YouTube channel about his condition and his hope to ward off the infection. Showing his personal example, he educated the people to follow precautions, healthy hygiene and practice Yoga to build immunity and face Covid-19 confidently.

After testing Covid negative, many people were heaving a sigh of relief, when the post Covid complications surfaced within a week to hospitalise him and lead to his eventual death.

The cruel Covid has once again taken away one of India's charismatic personalities who endeared himself to the film loving audience and to all their leading heroes, heroines, directors and producers, thus bridging the gap between their worlds.

Following passion, confidence in what you do and an ability to get along well with any person through an adaptive style and a humble demeanor, make TNR an unforgettable person with a permanent place on the online media and also in our hearts through the entertaining information he always provided us.

Like the many film personalities, TNR interviewed, we can try to emulate their success both on and off the film stage by learning and following their great deeds.

"A hero is an ordinary individual who finds the strength to persevere and endure in spite of overwhelming obstacles." – Christoper Reeve

CHAPTER 19: MR. SIDDHARTH SHRIRAM

"You only live once, but if you do it right, once is enough." — Mae West

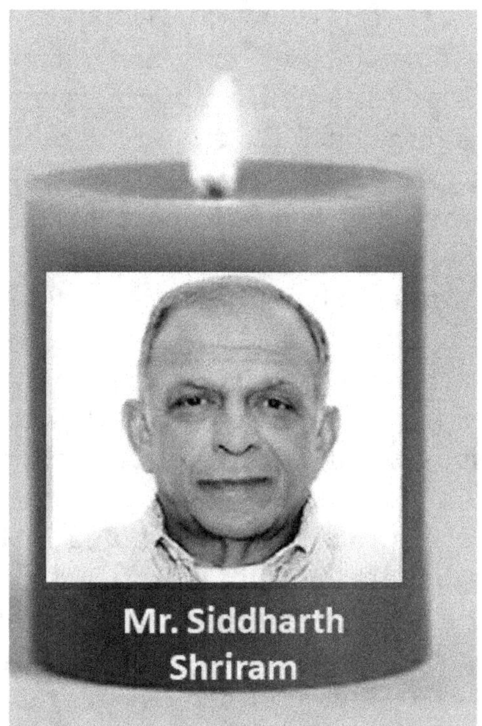

Siddharth Shriram (18.1.1945- 16.5.2021): Industrialist

Siddharth Shriram was one of the finest individuals and industrialists that India had till Covid took him away on the 16th of May 2021.

In many ways, Shriram sir led a dream life right from his birth till the very end. His zest for life, his approach to building international partnerships and his well-rounded personality with varied hobbies and interests makes his life a dream for anyone to lead.

Schooled in Welhem School and the Doon School at Dehradun,

graduated in English Literature from St. Stephens College, Delhi University, he completed his formal education at MIT, USA, as a Sloan Fellow with a Master of Science in Management.

He created joint ventures with Honda Motor Company to manufacture small engines and automobiles and was the Chairman of Honda Siel Cars India Ltd till recently.

Several sporting and healthful activities such as Golf/National Marathon/Frisbee. were sponsored by his companies under his leadership.

Despite being born into an extremely wealthy family, Siddharth Shriram, lived a life of discipline and went on to build solid foundations for a large business empire, without resting on the perks of richness. He was always focused on doing social work and investing in healthy activities on the corporate social responsibility front.

To empower women, Shriram sir focused on non-formal literacy programmes around his Mawana sugar factories; the Usha Sillai Schools, which train and give a machine and marketing collaterals to women in rural India to enable their self-employment, built around Usha's sewing machine business which exists in every state in India.

He wanted to play an active role in helping the country face the challenges through his NGO, Delhi Policy Group, a think tank that focuses on providing policy options to the government on a range of issues.

Till his life's end Siddharth actively participated in nation building dialog and at the same time led a fulfilling life by pursuing his interests in varied activities like Golf, Painting, Writing and mentoring large organisation.

While his loss is indeed a great void to fill, Siddharth Shriram's life can inspire many rich industrialists and their offspring's, not to rest on their laurels, but continue to strive for the society. The founders of new age companies, many of which are enjoying a quick rise to the unicorn status also can look up to the life of Siddharth Shriram to lead a well-rounded life while adding immense value to the society.

"No empire lasts forever; no dynasty continues unbroken. Someday, you and I will be mere legends. All that matters is whether we did what we could with the life that was given to us."
— Krishna Udayasankar.

CHAPTER 20: INSPIRING WOMEN WE LOST

She made broken look beautiful and strong look invincible. She walked with the Universe on her shoulders and made it look like a pair of wings."-Ariana Dancu

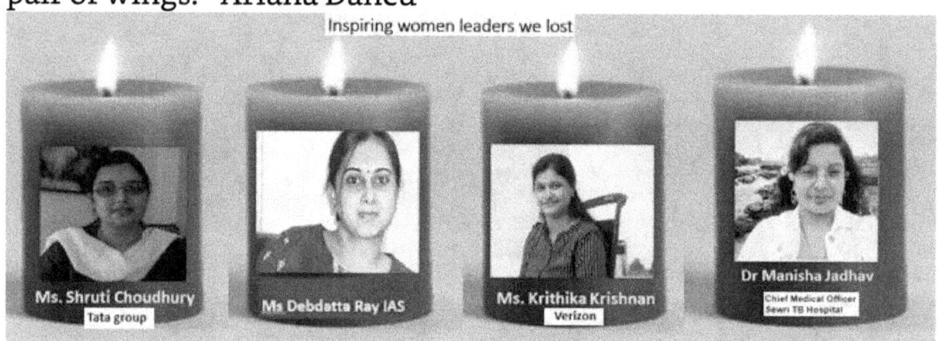

Women Leaders who left this world, a better place

Many great women leaders along with numerous doctors, nurses, frontline workers were snatched away from us, leaving a gaping hole in our society.

Shruthi Choudhury, Debdatta Ray, Krithika Krishnan, Dr. Manisha Jadhav are a few of the many amazing women who were at the forefront serving people both at office and in their family.

Women like these always inspired awe and admiration through their pursue of excellence at their work.

They also inspire the women all around who look upto them for motivation to achieve greater heights in their career.

Shruti Choudhury, alumnus of Xavier Institute of Social sciences was the Head HRM & Leadership development at Tata Steel, one of the outstanding Indian companies, when Covid-19 struck and took her away from this world. A senior member of the Tata family, as a head of the function that impacts most to the employees and their leaders, her loss leaves behind a major gap in the company, and also in the entire society which idolises its women leaders and gets inspired.

Krithika Krishnan is one of the rarest professionals in the Technology space. A senior women technologist, she always worked hard to inspire women in technology and spoke passionately about it in public events and forums. Known for her gentle, brilliant, no non-sense approach and great leadership skills, her passing away plunged numerous leading industry professionals and business associates into shock and sorrow.

Dr Debdatta Ray, a senior bureaucrat from West Bengal and Dr Manisha Jadha a senior Doctor and Chief medical officer at Sewri hospital are some of the precious souls who left us due to the Pandemic.

Dr Manisha Jadhav wrote in her Facebook post hours before her death, "Bodies die. Souls do not. Souls are immortal." Hope this holds good and they should return to Earth once again to continue their sojourn and to inspire all of us.

We rarely come across such gems of human beings and we hope the inspiration they leave behind will propel many more women to aspire and achieve greater success in the corporate world.

"Remember Red, hope is a good thing, maybe the best of things, and no good thing ever dies." Andy Dufresne, The Shawshank Redemption

CHAPTER 21:

Searching for Meaning & Inspirations amidst the Heartbreaks

"Hope is being able to see that there is light despite all of the darkness."- Desmond Tutu

The loss of so many amazing people is surely a cruel blow to all of us. Waking up every day during the peak of the pandemic was a scary event as we are not sure whom we will lose next. Covid-19 Pandemic was a secular disease which did not differentiate between people in any manner.

The people whom we lost and we commemorated in this book have left so much legacy, inspiring generations to come. Doing justice to them and their sacrifices means to learn from them and swear that we will lead our lives too to add value to the society and enjoy at the same time by living in the present to the fullest.

It is very important for us to understand that the tragedy is a short-term phenomenon and we should continue to rededicate our lives to the purpose we always set for ourselves.

Late Sir Victor Frankl, one of the greatest psychologists and researchers of human behaviour gives us great insights into how we can come understand (Book - Man's Search for Meaning) and to terms with the crisis through an approach named 'Logotherapy'.

According to Frankl, "We can discover the meaning in our lives in three different ways:

1. By creating a work or doing a deed;

2. By experiencing something or encountering someone; and

3. By the attitude we take toward unavoidable suffering" and that "everything can be taken from a man but one thing: the last of the

human freedoms – to choose one's attitude in any given set of circumstances".

To explain the nature of suffering and how we can come to terms with it, Sir Frankl gives the following amazing example, which can help us too, in these trying times.

"Once, an elderly general practitioner consulted me because of his severe depression. He could not overcome the loss of his wife who had died two years before and whom he had loved above all else. Now how could I help him? What should I tell him? I refrained from telling him anything, but instead confronted him with a question, "What would have happened, Doctor, if you had died first, and your wife would have had to survive without you?" "Oh," he said, "for her this would have been terrible; how she would have suffered!" Whereupon I replied, "You see, Doctor, such a suffering has been spared her, and it is you who have spared her this suffering; but now, you have to pay for it by surviving and mourning her." He said no word but shook my hand and calmly left the office.

The moral of the story is self-explanatory and left to the imagination of the readers. It is within us to come to terms with our sufferings and exercise our freedom to search for the meaning of our lives and repurpose or rededicate ourselves to achieve our potential and possibilities while enjoying every moment of this gifted life on earth.

"Hope is not the conviction that something will turn out well but the certainty that something makes sense, regardless of how it turns out."- Vaclav Havel

There have been many great persons who have helped us in channelising the energy of the people through yoga, exercise, dance, aerobics, nutrition etc., thus helping us in building a healthy lifestyle and string immunity system. These habits if followed and inculcated well, will stand us in good stead in the future too, while distracting us from the loss of our near & dear and of those whom we always looked upto.

"Let your hopes, not your hurts, shape your future."-Robert H.

Schuller

There have been many great personalities who inspired us through their actions and gave us hope and a reason to live and act. New trends have emerged, taken shape or accelerated that could transform our lifestyles forever. In the coming chapters, we shall look at some of the inspiring stories we discovered during the Pandemic.

Let us delve into some of these topics that offer us a hope and direct us to healthy future.

CHAPTER 22; Sonu Sood Messiah for the Migrants

"Could anything be better than this Waking up every day knowing that lots of people are smiling because you chose to impact lives, making the world a better place." Anyaele Sam Chiyson

If there is one famous person from the film industry, who has impacted most lives positively during the Pandemic, it is Sonu Sood, ironically well known for villain roles in the Indian cinema! He was indeed a real-life hero who has saved many lives and has been worshipped by many, who have benefitted from his great deeds.

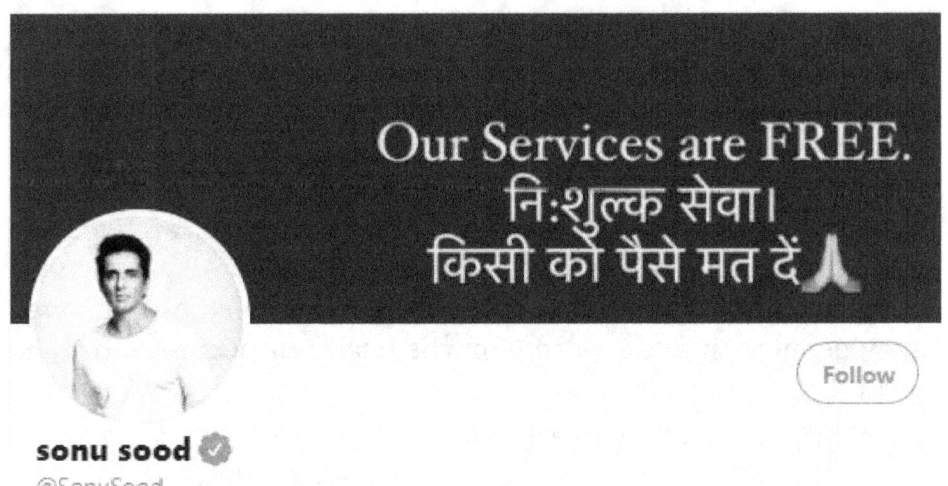

Sonu Sood: Immersed in serving the Humanity during the Pandemic

During the first wave of the Pandemic, when millions of migrant labourers had to leave their jobs and reach back to their home towns, they had to face many hardships, often going without food and earnings for many days at a stretch.

That is when he decided to do something to help the migrant workers and also a number of healthcare workers working day and night for the Pandemic.

"The power of one man or one woman doing the right thing for the right reason, and at the right time, is the greatest influence in our society."- Jack Kemp

Some of the steps that won the accolade from United Nations Development Programme in the form a Special Humanitarian award are recounted below:

1. Accommodating the Health care workers of Mumbai in his hotel in Juhu.

2. Serving food to over 45000 migrant workers every day through a program Shakti Annadanam in the name of his late father, Shakti Sagar Sood.

3. Helping over 20000 migrant workers to reach their home-

town by coordinating between them and the respective state governments,

4. Striving to provide employment to people through a special application PravasoRojgar.com

5. Arranging for Personal Protection Equipment to a number of front-line workers including Policemen and Healthcare workers serving the people in the time of Pandemic.

These are but many of the noble works he undertook and saved many people's lives and also won the hearts of people across the world.

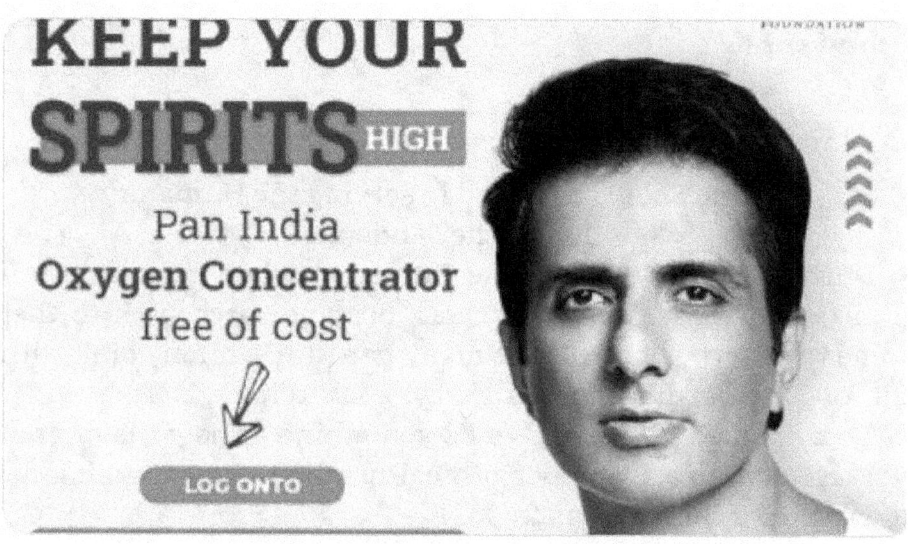

Sonu Sood: Reaching out Oxygen to the patients
across the country in time & free

When India was hit by the second wave of Covid from early March 2021, the hospitals were flooded with patients requiring Oxygen beds and ventilators. Sonu Sood once again swung into action to help the patients across the country to arrange free Oxygen concentrators at the door step of the needy patients through a national helpline. This was unprecedented at a time when the demand for the same was far exceeding the supply and the traders were resorting to hoarding the limited stock and selling them at exorbitant prices, fleecing the hapless patients, struggling to get their breath.

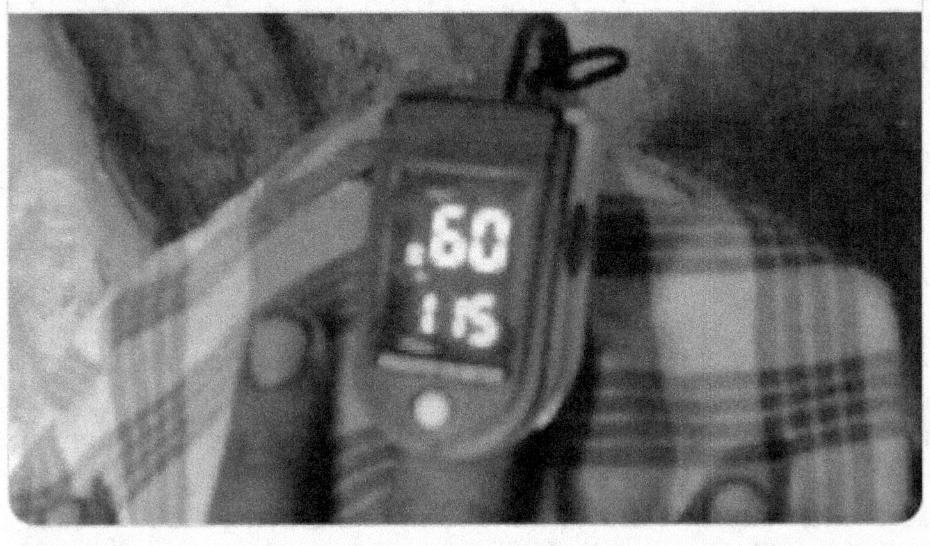

Sonu Sood turns the messiah for patients who required Oxygen concentrators

There have been several instances where the lives of patients across the country were saved due to the timely delivery of Oxygen concentrators in a miraculous manner.

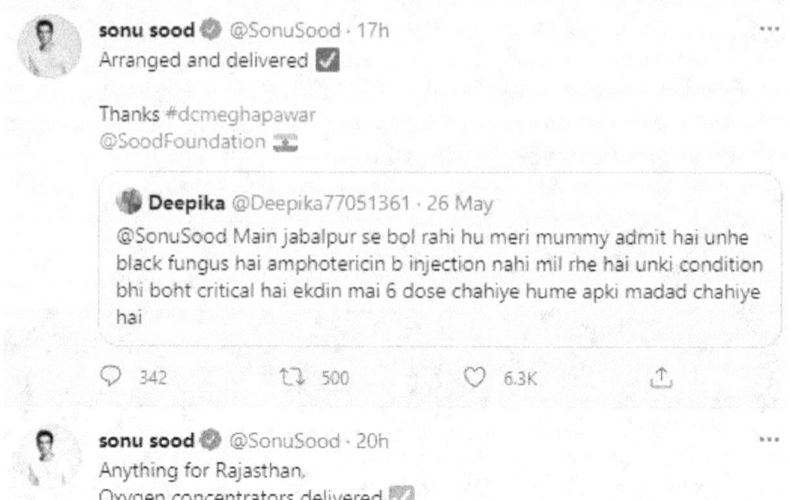

Sonu Sood as the go to man for every health care need in Pandemic

As the situation across the country worsened post the second covid wave, new diseases like black fungus infection, white fungus infection, yellow fungus infection started surfacing and threatened the lives of many patients. The sudden momentum of the dangerous life-threatening diseases caught the hospitals across the country off-guard and Sonu Sood with this national helpline and reach of his charitable infrastructure managed to help hospitals and patients get timely help in every case that came to his notice.

Through his noble acts Sonu Sood proved that one person with a good intention and make an enormous positive impact even in a large country like India.

"I am only one but still I am one. I cannot do everything, but still I can do something."-Edward Everett

Sonu Sood is definitely one of the greatest finds of the Pandemic and continues to inspire millions of people to think selflessly beyond their own little worlds and make a permanent place for themselves in the history of mankind.

"Some people arrive and make such a beautiful impact on your life, you can barely remember what life was like without them." Anna Taylor

CHAPTER 23:DR RANDEEP GULERIA

The Sage & The Savior

"In nothing do men more nearly approach the gods than in giving health to men."-- Marcus Tullius Cicero

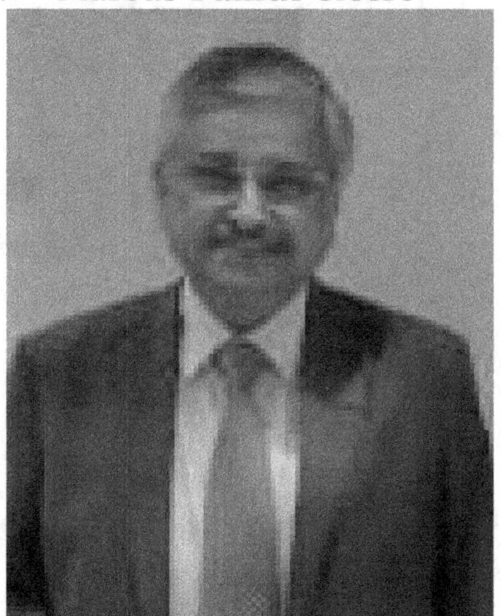

Padmashree Dr Randeep Guleria, Director AIIMS

If there is one person on the earth who has the power to save lives of millions of people and lead the country of a Pandemic successfully it is a great doctor who is also an excellent human being and efficient administrator at the helm.

India is fortunate to have one such person, Dr Randeep Guleria, the director of India's premier hospital, All India Institute of Medical Sciences, owned by the Government. Dr Randeep played a crucial role in managing the covid response across the country, in conjunction with Government of India during the Pandemic.

He has been awarded the prestigious Dr. B C Roy National Awards for the year 2014, under eminent medical person category by the Medical Council of India. He is regarded as one of India's leading medical expert.

Easily the best doctor India has ever seen (as experienced by myself, the author during a bout of sickness in 2013), Dr Randeep Guleria led the Government's efforts in a calm, composed and efficient manner to rein in the Pandemic that threatened to go out of control, many times due to the careless of the public and also the conduct of elections in many states.

He was omnipresent throughout the period across various TV channels, YouTube videos and write-ups in the media, guiding the medical fraternity, helping the government to focus its perspectives with well thought through and assessed opinions to formulate appropriate strategies and also cool the frayed nerves of the media and the people at large.

Working overtime and setting the right example by taking the vaccine doses when there was vaccine hesitancy all around, Dr Randeep Guleria was an epitome of perfection at the helm of the medical profession in India. Dr Guleria has been India's go to man to decode the various twists and turns of the pandemic times with the virus mutating often and new diseases like Black fungus and Yellow fungus emerging. Under his guidance, the government was able to take the rapid action needed to combat the virus and he was always present in the media bridging the much-needed communication needs with the medical fraternity through the media. This has gone a long way in reining back the things which at one point of time suddenly looked out of control when India was staring at a worst ever disaster following the reckless congregations across the county that led to this situation in the first place.

Under the able leadership of the government in Centre, it is indeed commendable that fantastic doctors like Dr Randeep have been given the right respect, role and responsibility in directing the country's efforts to rein in one of the deadliest Pandemics that posed innumerable challenges to the humanity. Surely lakhs of more lives would have been lost, but for the leadership provided by Dr Randeep Guleria. His presence at the helm, augurs well for the future of the country in managing the Covid-19 response across the country, in conjunction with Government of India during the Pandemic.

CHAPTER 24: MUKESH AMBANI
Covid Angel

"Creating a strong business and building a better world are not conflicting goals - they are both essential ingredients for long-term success."- Bill Ford

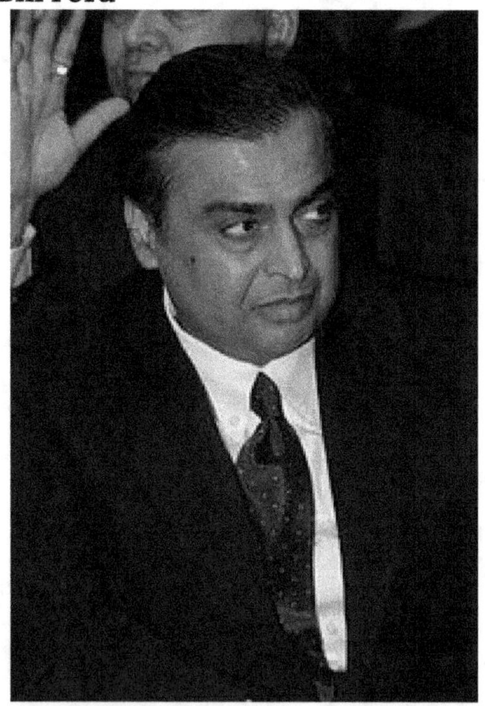

Mukesh Ambani: Chairman, Reliance Group

Reliance Industries is the largest publicly traded company in India with over two lakh employees and Market capitalisation of over Rs 14 lakh crores (close to 200 Billion US Dollars).

As Covid-19 Pandemic struck India, Reliance group. under the leadership of Mukesh Ambani helped the country fight the pandemic.

Some of the actions by Reliance group that can well be emulated by other organisations are as follows:

1. Donated over Rs 500 crores to PM Cares Covid relief fund.

2. Reliance has adopted a two-pronged approach to strengthen the availability of medical oxygen in India:

i. Refocusing several industrial processes at Reliance's Jamnagar and other facilities for rapid scale up in production of medical grade liquid oxygen. Reliance increased capacity to over 1000MT Medical grade Oxygen per day or over 11% of India's production and offered freely to over 1 lakh patients per day through various State Governments.

ii. Augmenting loading and transportation capacities to ensure its swift and safe supply to States and Union Territories across India. Airlifted 24 ISO containers to transport 500 MT oxygen per day across the country.

3. Six lakh employees belonging to RIL group companies viz., Reliance Foundation, Reliance Retail, Jio, Reliance Life Sciences, Reliance Industries contribute collectively to a Covid-19 action plan.

4. Opened a 100 bed-center set up at Seven Hills Hospital, Mumbai for Covid-19 patients. Special medical facilities are set tup to quarantine travelers from notified countries and suspected cases identified through contact tracing.

5. Manufactured over 1 lakh protective face masks per day as a part of PPE kits for medical staff

6. Provided 50 lakh free meals to the needy through non-governmental organisations (NGOs)

7. Provided free to emergency vehicles carrying Covid-19 patients through Reliance Petrol pumps.

8. Approved 5 years salary to be given to the family members of Reliance employees who lost their lives to Covid-19.

9. Free education till degree completion to all the children orphaned due to loss of parents to Covid-19.

These initiatives were very much the need of the hour and reflected the philanthropic nature of Asia's richest man, Mukesh Ambani, to help India come out of crisis. He is undoubtedly a Covid hero of India. Kudos to Mukesh Ambani and Reliance family to stand by and support the country setting an example to the corporate world.

CHAPTER 25: RATAN TATA
The model Corporate steward

"Ups and downs in life are very important to keep us going because a straight line even in an ECG means we are not alive."- Rata Tata, Tata Group

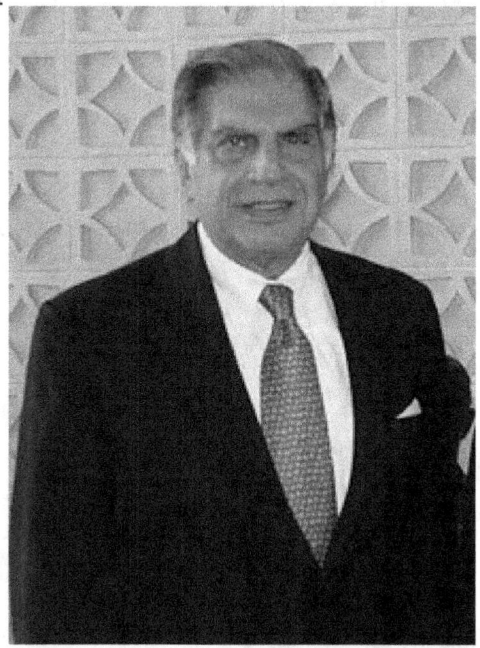

Padma Vibhushan Ratan Tata: Chairman, Tata Trusts

Iconic industrialist, philanthropist and Chairman of Tata Trusts, is one of the greatest Indian business leaders, who is known for ethics, integrity and positive attitude in business and for his philanthropy.

During the Covid-19 pandemic, Tata group and its charitable trusts under the guidance of Sir Ratan Tata, actively took part in the relief efforts in a number of ways, some of which are recounted below:

- Actively denounced any layoffs during the Pandemic, encouraging every company to prevent job losses, urging the companies to be sensitive and empathetic to the needs of their employees.

- Announced a special employee healthcare policy & lifetime salary of the Tata group company employees losing their lives to the nCovid19 virus, to the family members till the age of 60 of the deceased.

- Donated over 200 Million USD (over Rs 1500 crores) fron the group to PM's Corona relief fund.

- Sent over 200 tonnes of Oxygen daily to needy State Governments and Hospitals across the country.

- Provided 24 cryogenic containers to help transport oxygen across the country from manufacturing plants.

Ratan Tata always provided a sensible and empathetic leadership to all those associated with him and his group's activities. He always believed in taking every section of the society and his manpower together, hand in hand to conquer indomitable challenges.

"If you want to walk fast, walk alone. But if you want to walk far, walk together"- Ratan Tata

The kindness and empathetic nature of Sir Ratan Tata, one of the most successful Indians and a prominent face of the industry, goes a long way in healing the wounds caused by the Pandemic. Ratan Tata will continue to lead us and guide us many more years in the future as our true Hero.

CHAPTER 26: KAILASH SATYARTHI

The God of Children

"There is no greater violence than to deny the dreams of our children."- Kailash Satyarthi

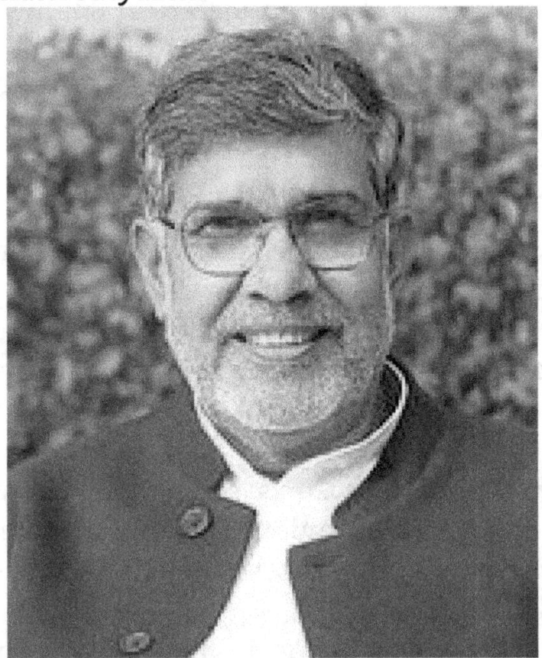

Kailash Satyarthi- Nobel Peace Laureate 2014

Covid-19 Pandemic destroyed many lives across the world. Over 10000 families in India lost both the parents orphaning their children in the Pandemic alone. While the children were spared from the death, the death of one or both the parents in many cases left the orphaned children with a life that is filled with sorrow, misery and depression. Only a messiah sent by God has the ability to rescue and guide the children who are faced with this unforeseen tragedy. India is blessed to have one such in the form of Kailash Satyarthi, a Nobel laureate recognised for his work in the area of children welfare.

Mr. Kailash Satyarthi is one of the tallest leaders and the loudest voice in the global fight against exploitation of children. Not caring even once about the life-threatening attacks that he has survived, Mr. Satyarthi has personally rescued tens of thousands of children from the scourge of slavery. His fearless and unrelenting policy advocacy efforts towards elimination of violence against children have resulted in path-breaking legislations globally.

He left a lucrative career as an Electrical Engineer and started 'Bachpan Bachao Andolan' (Save the Childhood Movement) to rescue children and their families from the shackles of slavery paving way for their reintegration into mainstream society with the help of state actors under the legal policy framework of India. Through his sustained policy advocacy efforts in India, he played a pivotal role in mobilizing support ensuring the passage of the Child Labour Act in the year 1986. Under the aegis of Mr. Satyarthi, Bachpan Bachao Andolan has rescued over 90,000 children from the scourge of bondage, trafficking and exploitative labour over the last four decades in India. (https://www.kailashsatyarthi.net/who-we-are).

India's Central and State Governments have announced plans to take of the children by providing them with financial support in the form of stipends and monthly pensions, free school admissions and education.

PM Modi said children who lost their parents to Covid-19 would get a monthly stipend once they turn 18 and a fund of ₹10 lakh when they turn 23 from PM-CARES

All children will be enrolled as a beneficiary under Ayushman Bharat Scheme (PM-JAY) with a health insurance cover of ₹5 lakh. (Source: Livemint)

However, the deep pain that the loss of the parents inflicts on the minds of the tiny tots is indeed unbearable and cannot be assuaged by provision of financial support and other superficial support. They need to be nurtured, comforted, guided and inspired to overcome the grief and achieve their potential and dreams.

There has to be a movement to adopt the children by well-meaning parents and the rescue homes for those not adopted or taken care by the relatives, should be well managed to ensure safe, secure lives to these children who need to be inspired and guided to live a life filled with purpose and fun.

The dreams of these young ones should never be allowed to be sacrificed and there is no better human being in India to ensure that the children of India, affected by the Pandemic to be taken care well throughout their lives to realise the dreams their parents had for their loved children.

Nobel Laureate Kailash Satyarthi & his foundation are the hope for India's Covid-19 orphaned children to enable them find a great future ahead.

CHAPTER 27: PRATIBHA AGARWAL

The Yoga Diva

"Yoga does not just change the way we see things, it transforms the person who sees." — B.K.S Iyengar

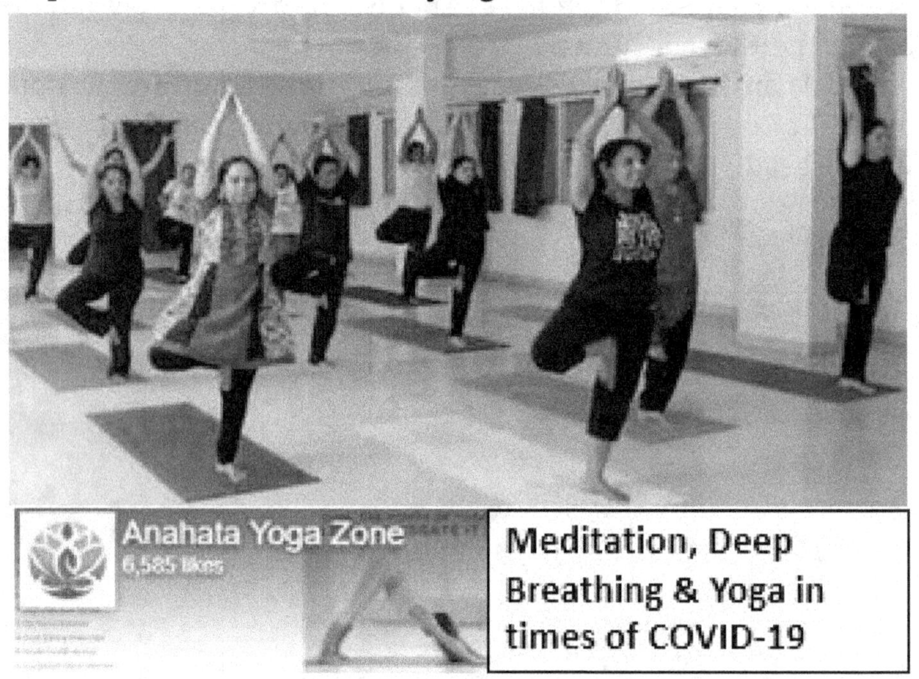

Anahata Yoga Zone: Hyderabad India
(https://www.anahatayoga.in/)

Covid19 is a disease aims at exploiting the weak immune system of the body & stress management is one of the key factors affecting the same. Thanks to Indian teachers and gurus like Swamy Baba Ramdev, Sri Sri Ravishankar, Sadhduru Jaggi Vasudev and Mahatriya (Ra), there has been a heightened awareness about the ancient Indian sciences like Yoga and Ayurveda to keep the human body's immune system fit and fine.

Anahata in Sanskrit, means "unhurt, unstruck, and unbeaten". Anahata Nad refers to the Vedic concept of unstruck sound (the sound of the celestial realm). Anahata is associated with balance, calmness, and serenity.

Prathibha Agarwal, the founder of Anahata Yoga Zone based out of Hyderabad India, is one of the finest exponents of Yoga across the world.

Yoga as exercise is a physical activity consisting mainly of postures, often connected by flowing sequences, sometimes accompanied by breathing exercises, and frequently ending with relaxation lying down or meditation. Yoga in this form has become familiar across the world, especially in America and Europe.

Being herself infected by Covid-19 in the early stages of the Pandemic, she helped healed herself, her family members and a number of patients she came across through Yoga and deep breathing exercises.

She took it upon herself to cure many people across the world through regular Deep breathing and meditation sessions, streamed live through her Facebook page. Termed Pranayama exercises for Covid healing, Ms Pratibha Agarwal has conducted many such sessions and for those who want to learn deeper about the topic, she offers very low priced and affordable short-term courses, that will enable them to make this activity, a part of their lives.

Pranayama that translates to 'regulation of life force energy' (prana) is the practice of breath control in yoga. In modern yoga as exercise, it consists of synchronising the breath with movements between asanas, but is also a distinct breathing exercise on its own, usually practiced after asanas. It involves a series of deep breathing exercises and other techniques that aim to control inhalations and exhalations, and sometimes include breath retention (kumbhaka). So, by practicing pranayama we are clearing the obstacles in our bodies, allowing breath and energy (prana) to flow freely. Our breathing is improved, our bodies function better and we clear and calm the mind.

The booklet given by NHS, UK offers a clear guidance about the types of breathing and physical exercises, Covid patients should undertake and it is available at the link: https://enderley.nhs.uk/wp-content/uploads/2020/04/Covid-booklet-post-discharge-hospital-FINAL.pdf .

If one wants to know more about Yoga and Meditation, you can follow Facebook page of Anahata zone, https://www.facebook.com/anahatayogazone.

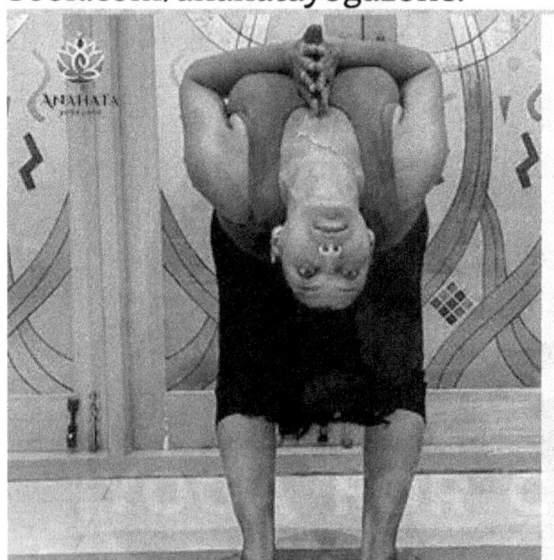

Anahata Yoga Zone: Globally Accredited
Teacher Training Programs

Anahata Yoga zone offers International Yoga Alliance's accredited teacher training courses that can enable anyone in the world to become successful trainers to spread this amazing practice that can heal & transform people into healthy souls.

"Meditation is silence, energising and fulfilling. Silent is the eloquent expression of the inexpressible. "– Sri Chinmoy (27 August 1931 – 11 October 2007), Indian spiritual leader who taught meditation.

Some of the important breathing techniques that Ms Pratibha taught through her numerous free classes include:

> 1. Anuloma Viloma , Pratiloma & Kumbhaka: Anuloma Viloma involves inhaling through both nostrils together and exhaling each breath alternately between the left and right

nostrils. The thumb of the right hand is used to manipulate the right nostril, while the pinky and ring finger are used to control the left nostril. Inverted Anuloma breath is called Pratiloma and involves inhaling through alternating nostrils and exhaling through both together. The practice of a kumbhaka or retention is encouraged as students advance at the practice; first at the end of the inhale and eventually the end of the exhale.

2. Bhastrika: Bhastrika is a kriya or 'cleansing action' along with kapalabhati to clear the airways in preparation for other pranayama techniques. Bhastrika involves a rapid and forceful process of inhalation and exhalation powered by the movement of the diaphragm.

3. Bhramari Pranayama: Bhramari (Humming bee breath) involves inhaling and exhaling by keeping index fingers on the ear's cartilage, releasing it while exhaling. A humming bee sound that is created while doing Bhramari and the exercise is known to increase the production of nitric oxide in the body by 15 times, resulting in a tremendous body resilience against the deadly coronaviruses.

4. Diaphragmatic Breathing: Diaphragmatic breathing, or "belly breathing," or abdominal breathing is designed to expand the lung capacity and is a much needed component of the treatment during nCovid19 infection. By pulling the diaphragm down while breathing inward, the Diaphragmatic breathing practitioner engages the stomach, abdominal muscles, and diaphragm. This technique is known to reduce heart rate, stress levels &

blood pressure and helps regulate the key processes in the body. It is a very key component of post trauma recovery process.

5. Kapalabhati (selectively used): Kapalabhati is a rapid breathing exercise that involves inhaling normally and exhaling rapidly in cycles, is very helpful in weight management & in reducing blood sugar levels, and stress levels. This is done selectively and not recommended in all situations especially for pregnant women and also sometimes for those suffering from Covid.

Ms Pratibha Agarwal can be considered as one of the greatest Covid heroes who has helped thousands of people to embrace the spirit of Yoga to improve their mind, soul & body functioning to beat the stress levels, make their lungs much healthier to face & beat the Covid-19 Pandemic

CHAPTER 28: DINAZ VERVATWALA

Keeping everyone in Shape

"Embrace each challenge in your life as an opportunity for self-transformation." – Bernie S. Siegel

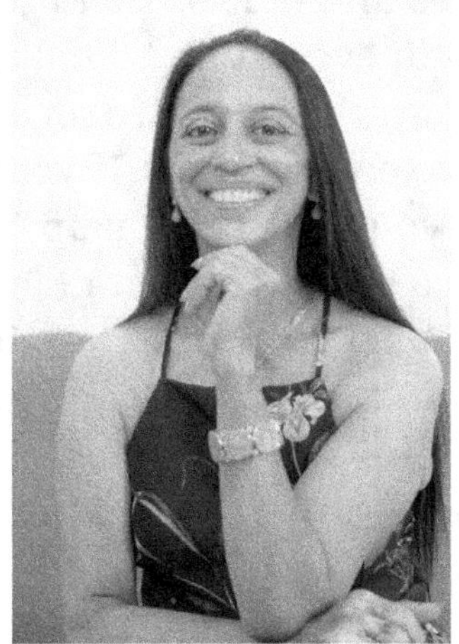

Dinaz Vervatwala: Guiness Record Holder for Aerobics

Covid-19 Pandemic made all the citizens of the world to focus on their fitness in an unprecedented manner, as a means to reduce co-morbidities like diabetes and heart problem, There is no better person than India's very own Guinness Record Holder, Ms Dinaz Vervatwala to channelise these activities into finely tuned programs that are easy to follow.

Stretch, Strength, Stamina and Stability are the four pillars of a perfect body and that is what Ms Dinaz Vervatwala, the globally renowned aerobics exponent and a fitness trainer par excellence, aims to achieve in every human being in the world.

With a mission to get every human being into a perfectly fit body frame, Ms Dinaz has touched the lives of lakhs of people across the world and transformed them beyond recognition, of course in a positive sense.

By driving every one of her students and followers beyond their comfort zone, Ms Dinaz made the pursuit of fit human body a fun filled activity with each of them motivating each other and egging them on to become fit.

If ever one wants to get into shape and stay there forever, all you need is to log once into her website https://dinazfitness.com/ and experience the action once.

Ms Dinaz Vervatwalla, is one amazing person who singlehandedly helped many people to become slim, attractive, confident and get rid of comorbidities and helped them to conquer Covid-19 & make the infection, an uneventful & trivial episode in their lives.

"You have to love yourself enough to set a standard for your life that you're unwilling to compromise. If you accept the standards of others for your life, you'll never be happy." – Tony Gaskins

Ms Dinaz Vervatwala sets highest standards for herself and all those come into her sphere, with a view to transforming their lives beyond recognition to become fit and fine for ever.

CHAPTER 29: DANCE WITH DEEPTI

Fitness through Entertainment

"To dance is to be out of yourself. Larger, more beautiful, more powerful… This is power, it is glory on earth and it is yours for the taking"- Agnes De Mille

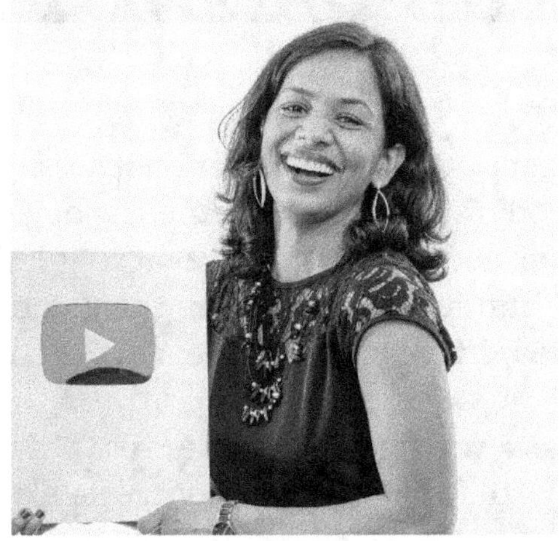

Dance with Deepti to Fitness- https:// www.dancewithdeepti.com/

Fitness through exercise and aerobics is the best way to tune up one's immune system and face diseases like Corona virus. What better way to exercise in the morning and the evening than through energizing and enjoyable dance?

A number of body builders and those exercise regularly at the Gymnasiums found it difficult to continue their activity due to the lockdowns and embargos in conduct of such centers, as the Covid-19 is deemed to be extremely contagious.

In such as scenario, it was the 'Workout at Home' that became the most popular pursuit to train the mind and body and keep fit & healthy.

Aerobics and choreographed dancing at home, offer a best way to burn excess body weight and tune up the muscle system and keep it string.

Ms Deepti, an amazing dancer and a personal fitness trainer captured the imagination of many people across the world through her YouTube channel, 'DancewithDeepti'.

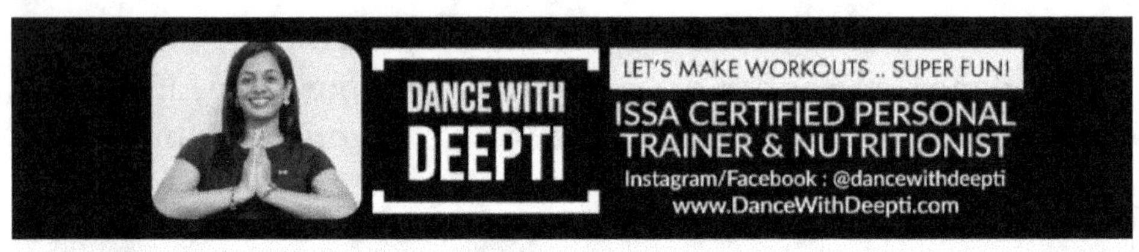

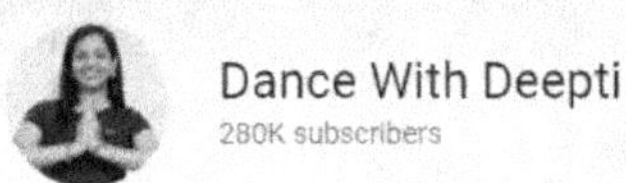

Dance with Deepti: Combine Fun and Fitness

Lockdowns and restricted movements have a tendency to make people lethargic and put on more fat that build more comorbidities into the human body, making them more vulnerable to Covid-19 and the best way to counter this is through immense physical activity.

One always has a resistance to undertake physical activity and if it is combined with fun and enjoyment, there is no better way to tune oneself up!

People discovered Dance with Deepti's channels and found it extremely enjoyable to follow the dances choreographed to burn fat and also tune muscles, while enjoying the music and the moves.

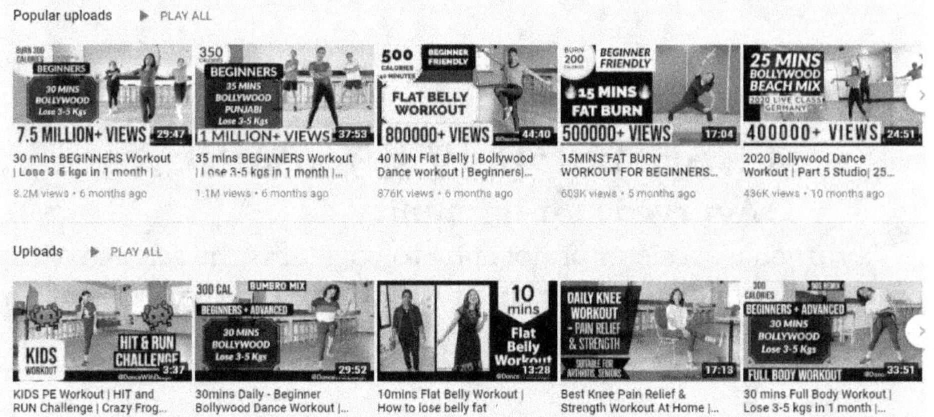

Fitness with Fun- Deepti's YouTube channel

Dances that simulate cardio exercises and also ABS workouts to strengthen body's muscles combined systematically and scientifically endeared Ms Deepti's channel to the people looking for ways and means to spend their lockdown times at home in a productive manner.

The popularity of fitness divas like Deepti, who have used their talents to spread joy, fitness, health and happiness has rightfully climbed up the charts and they are definitely the greatest finds during the Pandemic.

CHAPTER 30: BABA RAMDEV
Ayurveda for Immunity

"Ayurveda is a sister philosophy to yoga. It is the science of life or longevity and it teaches about the power and the cycles of nature, as well as the elements." ~ Christy Turlington

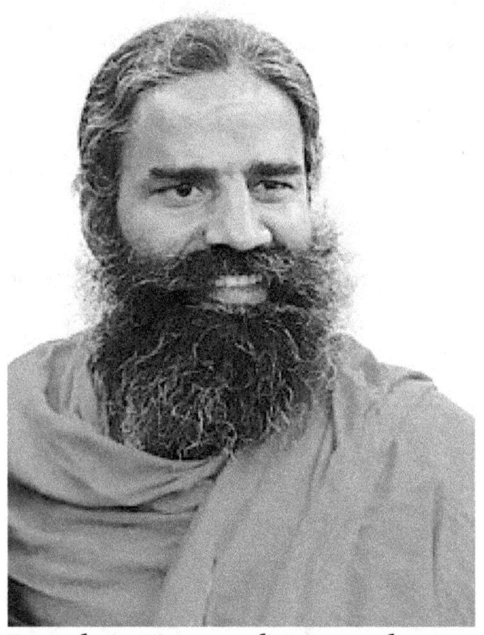

Baba Ramdev- Yoga and Ayurveda practitioner

Swami Ramdev (also known as Baba Ramdev) is an Indian Yogi, ayurvedic practitioner and businessman primarily known for his popularizing Yoga and Ayurveda in India. He is well known for his simple & frugal living and his passion to create low cost FMCG and healthcare supplements for Indians as an alternative to expensive products sold by the Multinational companies.

He is the one known as promoter of Indian heritage known as Ayurveda through a company Patanjali Ayurved Ltd., co-founded by him along with Acharya Balakrishna. His company rapidly grew to become one of the leading food & healthcare supplement product in India with an annual turnover of over Rs 5000 crores, employing over 2 lakh Indians, serving over 7 crore customers.

His product Coronil has helped India during the Covid crisis by helping Indians boost their immunity system Though there has not been claims that have been statistically proven to cure the coronavirus disease, this product has been recognized as an immunity supplement and has been used by many Indians who were suffering with Covid-19, with seemingly positive results. His contribution to the society in the form of promoting Ayurveda, creating jobs and Infrastructure has been commendable.

Ever since Covid-19 Pandemic started spreading its tentacles across India, Baba Ramdev has strived his best to put the best foot of its organization forward in finding a cure for the dreaded disease, as it was declared that Covid-19 has no known cure in allopathy. He was often at logger heads with the allopathy medical practitioners and Indian Medical Association, claiming that they are only good at misleading the patients without administering the right cure for the Covid-19 disease.

Though Swami Ramdev took back his allegations and negative remarks about the allopathic medical system, he managed to garner enough attention of all concerned to the importance of Ayurveda and meditation, the traditional Indian sciences and also was instrumental in the renewed focus on finding a cure and right line of treatment instead of fleecing the hapless patients with fat bills, despite the deaths in many cases.

The Covid-19 Pandemic has resulted in a renewed focus on traditional Indian sciences like Ayurveda, Yoga and Meditation exercised to build up the immunity system to fight such diseases better, thanks to efforts of Indian spiritual and ayurvedic gurus & practitioners like Swami Ramdev. He is definitely a great find as a result of the Pandemic.

CHAPTER 31: Natasha Mohan
Movement in Happiness

"Real transformation requires real honesty. If you want to move forward – get real with yourself." – Bryant McGill

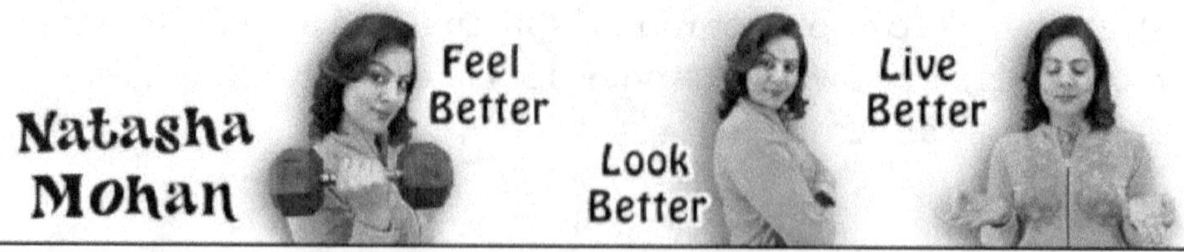

Weight loss with Natasha Mohan- YouTube channel
It is well known that excess body weight is the major cause for a

lot of comorbidities in a human being that makes one susceptible to death in case of Covid-19 infection.

This is where iconic wellness experts who combine a number of facets of human wellbeing by integrating right quality & quantity of food & exercise strive to propagate.

"He who has health has hope, and he who has hope has everything." – Arabian Proverb

Natasha Mohan, after year and years of working with food, and lots of research, came up with the best Indian diet plan coupled with right type of exercising one's body needs to lose weight. By making sure our body gets the right amounts of all important source to energy and vitamins while burning excess calories & maintaining muscle strength, Ms Natasha Mohan achieves excellent results in a healthy body weight loss. Starting by experimenting and perfecting the techniques on herself with stupendous results, she has now impacted lives of millions of Indians positively, leading them to a healthy & happy life, rid of life-threatening comorbidities.

Ms. Natasha Mohan's YouTube channel 'Weight Loss with Natasha Mohan' is a highly followed social media outposts by lakhs of health-conscious viewers. In times of Pandemic caused by diseases like Covid-19, her impact on the society in reducing the mortality amongst the patients is indeed commendable. She is one of the best and noteworthy finds of the Pandemic times.

CHAPTER 32: Rujuta Diwekar
Goddess of Nutrition

"This is what people don't understand: obesity is a symptom of poverty. It's not a lifestyle choice where people are just eating and not exercising. It's because kids – and this is the problem with school lunch right now – are getting sugar, fat and empty calories – but no nutrition." – Tom Colicchio

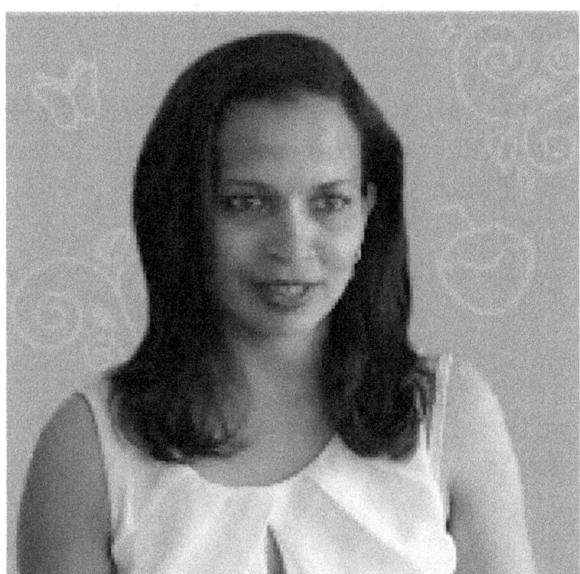

Rujuta Diwekar: India's Most loved nutritionist

Immunity is the weapon with which a human body fights disease like Covid-19.

Nutrition is the most important factor in building a human's immunity system. Rujuta Diwekar, India's foremost nutrition expert and a well acknowledged author in this domain has been providing yeomen service in educating and disseminating a lot of information to people across the world.

Through her Youtube channel 'Rujutadiwekarofficial', Ms Rujuta explains to the audience about what to eat, how much to eat and how to cook for a healthy body that always looks fresh and active.

Healthy diet, optimal exercise and a good sleep are the right ingredients for a perfect immune system.

Follow these golden rules and it is very difficult for a Coronavirus or any co-morbid diseases like Blood pressure, Diabetes and many others to come anywhere near causing trouble to you.

Pandemic helped people rediscover the importance of right nutrition and Rujuta Diwekar with her emphasis on teaching the same to the people, free of cost, is the right medicine the God ordered for India during such times. She is undoubtedly one of the great finds, India uncovered during the Covid-19 pandemic, to become a national treasure.

"The doctors of the future will no longer treat the human frame with drugs, but rather will cure and prevent disease with nutrition." – Thomas Edison

CHAPTER 33: TEJASVI SURYA
Leading from the front

The task of the leader is to get his people from where they are to where they have not been.

Henry Kissinger

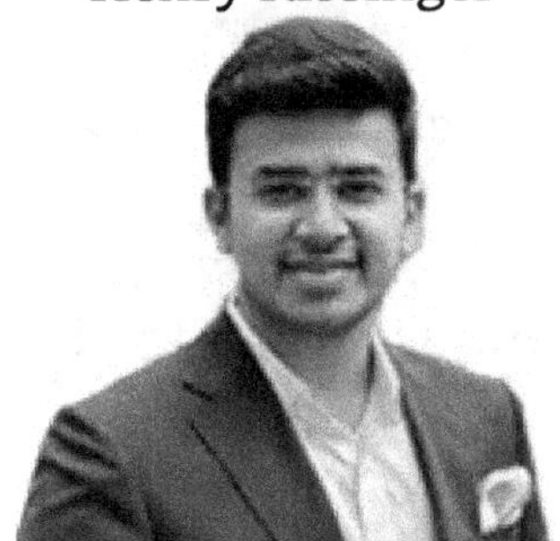

Tejasvi Surya: Messiah for Covid Patients
and Member of Parliament

Covid-19 Pandemic swept the country off its balance, outing millions of people and their families into distress, helplessness, poverty and depression. The Government and the medical machinery of the country was in often in disarray and it took time for it to get a grip of the situation even if it took rapid action on multiple fronts.

India required its politicians and its Government officials led by its able and dynamic leaders to reach out to the citizens and coordinate the actions on all fronts. This is easier said than done, when everyone was also trying to shield themselves away from this dreaded and contagious disease. Most of them have been waiting to come out into open after the Pandemic ends.

Fortunately, there are leaders like Tejasvi Surya, a dynamic and young parliamentarian who is working like a foot soldier, sacrificing his comfort and declared a war on the Pandemic to support the citizens on multiple fronts.

Tejasvi took several proactive steps to ensure that the benefits of the various Government programs are reaching the needy. He tried to ensure that the covid patients are able to reach to the required care and are provided accurate and timely information. He also created a covid helpline and is coordinating free vaccination camps and aid to the needy.

Exposing the irregularities in allocating beds in Covid hospitals, Tejasvi Surya differed with his own party men and ensured that favoritism and partiality of any kind is not done that denies needy patients to get the right care at hospitals.

He leveraged technology to the hilt and operated Covid helplines to give accurate information to the citizens about the availability of beds, Oxygen and other medical resources. He also worked alongside his party and team members to ensure availability of free medical supplies to the needy patients thus saving a lot of lives.

During the time of the lockdowns citizens faced severe problems in getting household supplies and Tejasvi and his followers operated online delivery system of essential items to address this problem.

The service can be easily used by citizens using basic handsets too, as they can reach out to the helpline number to place orders verbally. Citizens could place specific requirements (including brand name of products) and the required quantity. Delivery executives would ensure that each user's needs are met within 24 hours," Surya said.

During the Pandemic, Tejasvi was one of the most familiar political faces educating the public about the dangers of coronavirus, importance of adhering to social distancing and covid guidelines and most importantly, the need for everyone to be vaccinated.

Though he was trolled by the opposition parties for his animated approach and passionate approach to whatever he does, Tejasvi kept his cool and continued to work aggressively to ensure free covid vaccination to poor people who cannot afford, educating the people to minimize the spread of the pandemic, ensuring availability of beds to the patients and dissemination of the information to all and also highlighted the plights of the children orphaned due to the loss of their parents to this dreaded disease.

Through his acts, Tejasvi Surya gave hope and inspiration to the crores of citizens of India. He signaled a message that, those in power need not be sitting in ivory towers, but can risk themselves and be omnipresent to fight for the welfare of the people, even in a contagious pandemic, provided they adhere to the laid-out norms.

Tejasvi Surya is undoubtedly a model politician and a great hope for the citizens of this country, especially the youth. His pro-active work during the Pandemic will remain unparalleled and be forever etched in the minds of the thankful citizens of Karnataka, India.

CHAPTER 34: KRISHNA ELLA
Atma Nirbhar Vaccine

"Although our main concern is to treat people with substance use disorder and mental health issues and to ultimately prepare them for reintegration into society, vaccination is crucial in terms of ensuring overall health and well-being."- Susanne Bjelbo, nurse and social worker.

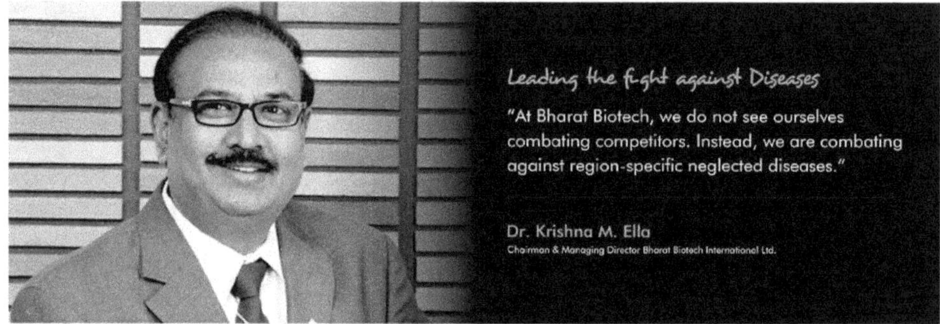

Dr. Krishna Ella: Leading India's Vaccination drive

Vaccination is the best tool to reach herd immunity against the Pandemic that spreads across the population in the country like a wild fire. The vaccines also have to be affordable for a developing country like India that needs to vaccinate a billion citizens.

It is easier said than done, as it takes decades & a very huge investment to come out with vaccines against any new disease. Further, they have not seen successful vaccination programs against diseases caused by Coronavirus group of viruses. In other words, India was fighting a hopeless battle to overcome a tragedy, against very high odds.

Fortunately, India has Bharat Biotech, a company founded by Dr Krishna Ella and Dr Suchitra Ella along with their able team, that empowered the country to fight an invisible powerful enemy and push it back in its tracks. Dr Krishna Ella, overpowered many setbacks and naysayers who gave little chance of success in this crusade to save the population undoubtedly inspired and led his company to become a greatest saviour of humanity through their vaccine, 'Covaxin' that has proved effective against many strains. This was done when there was a sense of disbelief, leave alone opposition from people who spread doubt and distraction against the efforts to create vaccines in the very first place.

"The ultimate measure of a man is not where he stands in moments of comfort and convenience, but where he stands at times of challenge and controversy." – Martin Luther King, Jr.

Dr. Krishna Ella is the Chairman & Managing Director of Bharat Biotech International Limited, which he incorporated in 1996. A gold medalist at university, Dr. Ella worked as a research faculty at the Medical University of South Carolina, Charleston after earning his Ph.D. from the University of Wisconsin-Madison. A research scientist in Molecular Biology, Dr. Ella strongly believes that innovative technology in vaccine development is essential to solve public healthcare problems caused by infectious diseases. Under Dr. Ella's leadership, Bharat Biotech has grown to become a global leader in innovative vaccine.

When Covid-19 struck and the Pandemic started spreading faster than the speed of thought, Dr Krishna Ella, well experienced in the art of creating affordable vaccines, realised that the vaccines should not just be safe and effective, but also practical. When the rest of the world went for cutting edge mRNA tech, Dr Krishna experimented with the killed virus vaccine, developed in association with ICMR (Indian council for Medical Research, a Government of India undertaking).

With the support from ICMR, the regulatory body - the company was able to accelerate the whole process of pre-clinical studies and got into human testing in a few months. With approval from ICMR, Bharat Biotech converted its India's biggest BSL-3 high-containment facility for manufacturing inactivated polio vaccine to manufacture COVID-19 vaccine. This became a success, giving India it's very own affordable & effective vaccine at double quick time.

Thus, Dr Krishna Ella rose from the humble beginning as a

farmer's son to become a scientist who helped India face up to the biggest and indomitable challenge that threatened lives of millions of its citizens. India asserted its place once again in the world map as a vaccine superpower, this time not just in value for money products, but also as a pioneering researcher.

"I haven't got any (Bill & Melinda) Gates Foundation money, I have not got any money from (the) government of India, I have taken all the risk of creating a BSL-III facility, we have done clinical trials at our own cost, and manufactured 20 million doses at risk, I never said the government should buy, It's the moral responsibility as a scientist that I should do for the country," Dr Krishna Ella said, addressing his detractors in a Press conference in January 2021.

Afterall, "A truly strong person does not need the approval of others any more than a lion needs the approval of sheep." said, Vernon Howard

Launched in a record time, Covaxin, Bharat Biotech, Dr Ellas and their team are the greatest finds of the Pandemic times and have etched their names forever in the annals of India's history.

CHAPTER 35: VENTILATOR PROJECT BREATH FOR INDIA

"Against all odds, a seed rises from darkness and beautifies the universe."
— Matshona Dhliwayo

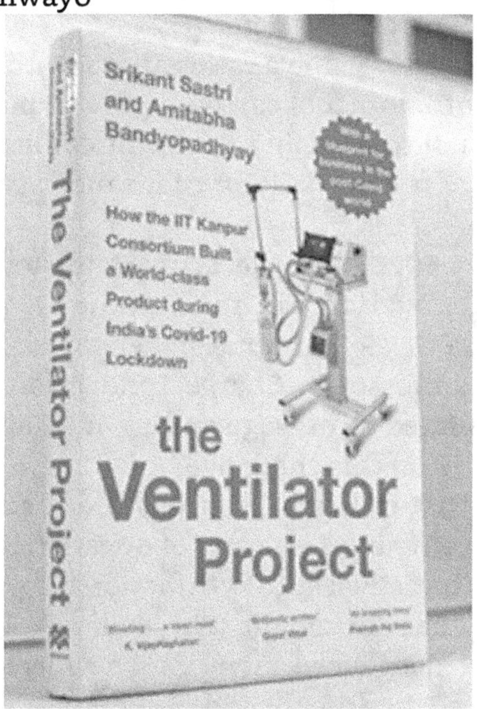

The Ventilator Project at IIT Kanpur: https://
www.iitk.ac.in/new/the-ventilator-project

Covid-19 has been found to lower the oxygen level in the affected human's body and supplementing the body's efforts to breath in oxygen has become a necessary part of the covid treatment protocol. As per WHO, Optimal supportive care includes oxygen for severely ill patients and those who are at risk for severe disease and more advanced respiratory support such as ventilation for patients who are critically ill.

Ventilators are normally used in hospitals on patients in very selective and thus rare life-threatening situations and hence the stock of such devices across the entire hospital network is always limited and definitely no-where in scale to manage the demand created by a Pandemic like Covid-19.

High cost of Ventilators and difficulty in making medical grade high quality equipment meant that, not only patients had to be prepared with heavy bills due to high daily charges of the ICUs, but also the country had to shell out enormous amounts of precious foreign exchange importing them.

This meant that it became a necessity for India to develop low cost-effective Ventilators that can be approved, manufactured and distributed in double quick time across the country to manage the patients getting admitted daily in thousands across the country into the ICUs.

On 16th March 2020, Hon'ble Prime Minister, Shri Narendra Modi, released the clarion call for battling COVID-19 with the launch of the COVID-19 Solution Challenge. Professor Amitabha Bandyopadhyay Professor-in-Charge, Innovation and Incubation, IIT Kanpur, circulated a message among IIT Kanpur's incubated companies to work on this challenge.

The result of that call, galvanized by the sheer grit and ambition of one such company, Noccarc Robotics, led Nikhil Kurele and Harshit Rathore to deliver a fully-functional low-cost ventilator amidst a nationwide lockdown. The courageous entrepreneurs were backed by experienced mentors who made the impossible happen in 90 days. They met over daily Zoom calls and exchanged WhatsApp texts to overcome the unforgiving lockdown restrictions. Since then, the Noccarc team has been a proud recipient of numerous accolades, the most recent being the winner at the India International Science Festival (IISF, 2020) in the 'ventilator' category.

Prof Amitabha and Prof Srikant Sastry captured the inspiring story about how academic institutions entrepreneurs and industry to collaborate more closely for making India achieve leadership status in technology development.", in their book depicted in the above figure, namely, 'The Ventilator Project.'

The project resulted in fulfilling the burgeoning demand of this extremely critical medical product, when it was needed most, finding its way to hospitals across the country treating Covid patients.

The Ventilator Project by IIT Kanpur incubators is definitely one of the best finds of the Pandemic and reinforces our faith in the ability of India to become a leading manufacturers of high technology products in the future, by leveraging the collective talent of its great institutions and the promising startup ecosystem.

CHAPTER 36: 2-DG,
ANTI COVID DRUG
Made in India Medicine: 2-DG

"Our greatest glory is not in never falling, but in rising every time we fall."-Confucius

Indian scientists declared a major breakthrough in their fight against nCovid-19 virus, when Drug Controller General of India gave an emergency approval to an anti-cancer formulation-based therapeutic application,

2-Deoxy-D-glucose to treat patients in advanced stage of infection.

This anti-covid formulation was developed in Institute of Nuclear medicine and allied Sciences (INMAS), a lab of India's premier Government owned Research organisation, DRDO and India's leading pharmaceutical company, Dr Reddy's Labs, Hyderabad. showed perceptible results in early trials to dramatically cut down the growth and multiplication of the virus by selectively starving the virus cells of oxygen, while supporting the damaged body cells. The drug comes in sachet and is convenient to administer orally in water dissolvable powder form. The drug was fast-tracked and given approval on 8th of May 2021.

In the first week of June 2021, '2-deoxy-D-glucose' was administered successfully in a few hospitals and led to the recovery of serious patients in ICUs and on ventilators. It reduced the dependency of the patients on external Oxygen support, increased their SPO2 levels above the threshold in 2-3 days facilitating their discharge from the ICUs, quickly.

The speed with which Indian Government has facilitated a new break through drug to reach the market and save lives, shows the coming of age of the country in leveraging cutting edge science and technology expertise to save the lives in critical situation.

This new found expertise and execution excellence has been a great find during the Pandemic times and augurs well for India to become a global leader in Medical & Pharma domains in the future.

CHAPTER 37: WFH & BFM

Going Digital

Work from home and Buy from Mobile became the new normal during the Covid era that started early 2020 and continued throughout the Pandemic period. This has led to an unprecedented boom in consumption of everything 'Digital' that also led to a rapid Digital Transformation across Governments & Organisations.

The Covid Pandemic led to movement restrictions for citizens across the world including complete lockdowns, that affected the ability of households to procure essential products and services. With Governments across the world relaxing the movement restrictions for supply chain and household delivery of essential products, there has been an unprecedented and unforeseen growth in the digital and e-commerce sectors. Thus, a migration to ecommerce-based services across the world has been a significant outcome of the COVID-19 crisis. Consumers on their part adapted to the lockdowns which were becoming a new normal by becoming 'Digital' and consuming most of the products and services they needed, through their mobile and laptops.

As per OECD, significant increases were observed for food services (over 60%), household goods (close to 50%) and food & beverages, pharmaceutical products, including medicines and mobile & online based payment services across the globe.

The routine for a household shifted from consuming offline services and buying in physical outlets to doing everything from the comfort of their homes. Some of the key activities that went mostly online are:

1. Gym, Yoga, Meditation and fitness related activities guided by online instructors.

2. Online meetings including birthday & other

occasional celebrations as against house visits & physical parties and get togethers

3. Buying all household goods, medicines, food & beverages and all other consumer goods through ecommerce portals & food delivery apps,

4. Online webinars and trainings instead of classroom-oriented teaching,

5. Official meetings, conferences and discussions through video conferencing and above all

6. Watching movies, plays and other entertainment content over OTT channels like Amazon Prime, Netflix, ZEE5, YuppTV, SunDirect etc.

UNCTAD Acting Secretary-General Isabelle Durant observed that, the quick adaptation of both businesses and consumers to dealing digitally with each other cushioned the economic impact of the lockdowns, shielding global economies from a downturn.

"They have also sped up a digital transition that will have lasting impacts on our societies and daily lives – for which not everyone is prepared," she said, adding: "Developing countries should not only be consumers but also active players and thus producers of the digital economy."

A highly contagious disease that Covid-19 led to imposition and observation of movement restrictions with government-imposed Lockdowns becoming a norm. The resultant shift of consumption of a variety of products & services to online, also leading to a disruptive digitally transformative trends, is one of the striking finds of the Pandemic.

TRANSFORMATION JOURNEY DURING THE PANDEMIC

"Just when the caterpillar thought the world was ending, he turned into a butterfly." —Anonymous proverb

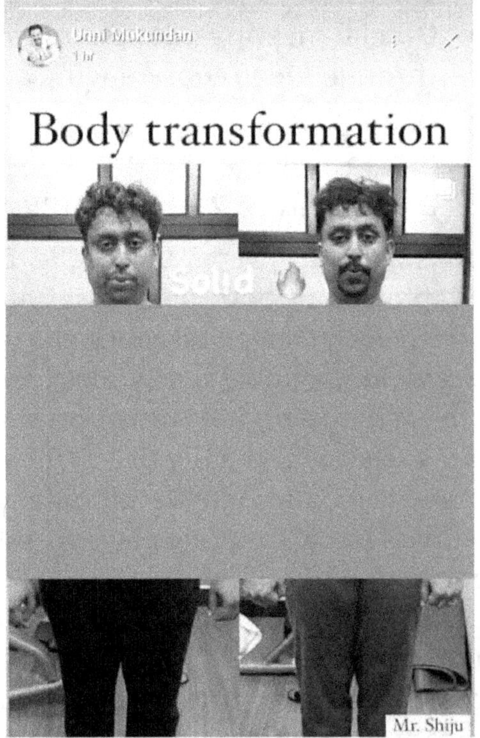

Shiju MV- Inspiring Body transformation

In this chapter, I would like to recount the story of Shiju MV, my ex-colleague at ULTS, Kozhikode Kerala, now working as a lead assistant manager at ULTS. While the Lockdowns inflicted lack of physical movement for most of the citizens advised not to move out in the open, there was a possibility of bodies growing obese and unhealthy to breed more comorbidities. The depressing news of death and sickness carried in abundance by the media channels also resulted in pent up frustration and despair leading to mental health problems for many. A case in point is the withdrawal of the World Champion Tennis player Osaka from French Open Tennis championship on 1ˢᵗ June 2021, owing to stress and mental health situation.

It is important for everyone in such a situation to continuously repurpose themselves challenging their mind and body with new interesting goals leading to a healthy mental and physical life.

Shiju is one such person, who channelised his energies and transformed himself from an Obese and slow-moving individual (though with a great sense of humor and heart of gold) to a lean, attractive and confident human being with a great physique. This is not just an isolated effort. There have been many such cases of inspiring journey of transformation through the lockdowns, People found new pursuits whether they or of literary, cultural, spiritual, educational, sports, philanthropy or physical dimension with a new found vigour to transformation.

Here is the story of Shiju's transformation, in his own words!

One small virus has changed the outlook of the world, similarly, one small positive thought can change our mind towards leading a lifestyle that we want. Health came out to be the most important and the top priority in today's new normal. Be it the immune system, diet, eating healthy etc. each one of us was looking towards a healthy lifestyle free from any disease and maintain that strength to fight against this lethal virus.

My quest towards reshaping my body was my gift to me on my birthday. It was not a drive towards building up huge muscles, it was a desire to get fit and aimed at feeling good. In November 2020 which happens to be my birthday month, I decided to give myself the gift of being a healthier me. As per all the resolutions that we take, we tend to deviate ourselves but how do you ensure you don't lose focus? Now, I took a look at how far I have come and how hard I have worked for my current physique. I realized that I don't want all of it to go to waste & do better than what I did the previous day. This kept me focused. I started with cardio exercises moving to weights. Cardio and bodyweight exercises are good to maintain your muscle mass, but will even burn more calories, decreasing your body fat percentage quicker.

In addition to eating healthy, it is also important to eat the right amount. It is important to understand that losing weight is all about replacing your unhealthy cravings with the right food. I made fitness, eating healthy a part of my daily routine and also started drinking more water.

Approximately after 4 months, I got my gift and it was a huge surprise as well. Mr Unni Mukundan, a Malayalam cine actor selected my picture for being able to transform and getting fitter. I was not aware of the Instagram status being put by him. As a surprise to me, one of our colleague Mr Vishnu Prakash from the Creative Media team shared his Instagram post with me. I was thrilled that my efforts paid off and I was able to get featured and inspire others as well.

We still do not know how the virus will play out and nobody is sure how things will be in the coming months, so, this time around let us invest to make ourselves more productive, enhanced, balanced & competent. We need to incline ourselves and get fitter and healthier by upgrading and enhancing our faculties.

My wish to all is to pursue a healthy life and in turn pursue happiness! ... Shiju MV

I sincerely hope that many more people find such joyful and healthy pursuits to transform their bodies and souls and enjoy their post Pandemic lives.

"Life isn't about waiting for the storm to pass...It's about learning to dance in the rain." Vivian Greene

INSPIRATIONS FOR THE FUTURE

What strengths and talents can you repurpose for a new endeavor? How can you re-purpose your thoughts to ensure they help you rather than hinder?" — Susan C. Young

Covid-19 Pandemic has taught us many lessons. It has created a new found immunity in our bodies through the many good and transformative habits we inculcated along with an improved hygiene outlook.

We have faced many heartbreaks and many have now lost a sense of emotion to the extent that there is nothing to be broken. However, we need to continue to live and lead purposeful lives. Taking the lives of those who lost their lives to Covid-19 pandemic but continue to touch people's lives by inspiring them through their lingering fragrance filled lives gives us some pointers to how we can continue to repurpose ourselves and push ourselves up from here.

One of the finest activities to work on is to start something new or create a new enterprise itself. Entrepreneurs and Startups like Rajeev Karwal, have set a great example and inspired many enterprises to follow pathbreaking ideas and create ventures offering enormous value to society & created livelihood opportunities to many. There is nothing more satisfying than impacting so many lives positively.

The ikigai principle helps us in following our hearts to do the most productive and profitable activities. When we undertake any activity that is in line with our passion it will yield the best results. But there is more to it. We need to consider the following factors before setting out on any new project.

1. Do what you love &are passionate about.

2. Focus on doing the things you good at it. If not strive to develop your acumen in it.

3. Important to do things that lead to addition of value to the society and all those around to ensure that you get paid for it.

4. It is imperative to focus on activities that are good for the society and to the environment.

The above factors help us to focus our activities in the right direction.

The book 'Dhool Dhoop Dhakka' by my friend Deepak Ghadge and Arun lal, gives the important factors for success of any new venture.

The PHD factor namely Passion for activity, Hunger for achievement and Disciplined approach are the right ingredients for an entrepreneur's success and when channelised in the right direction in line with the 4 points outlined above, the effect will be gratifying and everlasting creating sustainable ventures.

"Nothing great in the world has ever been accomplished without passion." – Georg Hegel

The great people we have seen in this book have followed some are all of the below mentioned criteria to channelise their actions in normal situations too for maximum impact. When you undertake any activity, please consider:

- Is it a requirement?

- Is it a must do?

- Is it profitable to invest time and resources in it?

- Can we pull it off within our organizational means?

- Is it noteworthy and referred fondly by people?

- If it good for the society and the environment?

- Can we get the right staff to be able to deliver the project 100%?

- Can we take care of our employees and service our assets in the long run?

Great actions when repeated over long periods in a sustainable manner have the ability to create a long term value to the society and capture the hearts of the people. People who enjoy doing and have excelled in whatever they undertake whether, as an entrepreneur or as an individual employee, doctor, politician, public servant or a theatre artist will spread joy all those around. Such people will continue to inspire us and have the potential to capture their place in our hearts forever. This also should be the goal for us.

Yes, we have lost in Pandemic, many great persons and angelic souls that have found their lasting peace in the abode of God,

We also Found in Pandemic many heroes and new approaches to life and a new found inspiration to carry on the legacy of all those who left us for a greater future.

We should always remember what Late Stephen Hawking, one of the greatest Human beings ever lived said, "If there's life, there is hope." -Stephen Hawking.

Let us work to continue the good work and make way for a better way when the souls that we lost to the Pandemic make way back to this world through their rebirth. Hopefully we have a way to recognise them, by then!

ABOUT THE AUTHOR

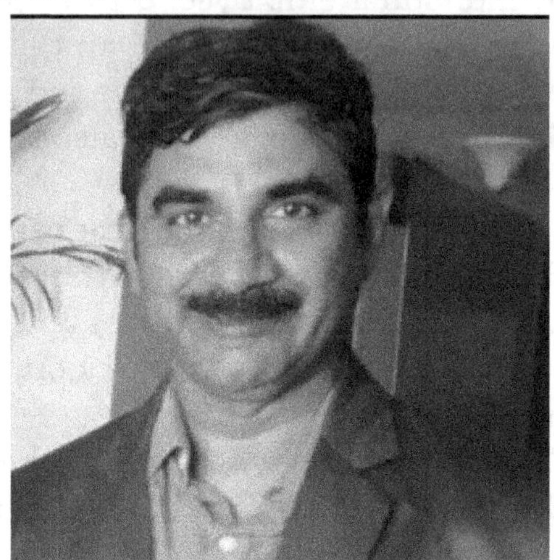

Srinivas Mahankali: Author- Corona Wars

Srinivas Mahankali is an alumnus of IIT Madras and IIM Bangalore and has served as Head of Blockchain & Emerging Centers of Excellence in Government and Private Organisations. He is certified in Lean Six Sigma, NCFM Level 2, Capital Markets and R3 Corda & IBM Microservices and Digital Marketing. He has worked as CXO./ CIO in leading organisations.

His book 'Decoding Innovation- Modelling the 21st Century Enterprise' delves deep into the scale-up strategies for start-ups with potential to become exponential organisations.

He has authored and co-authored two prominent books 'Blockchain–The Untold Story' and 'AI & ML Powered Agents of Automation and Successful Organisations in Action', respectively, his book 'Blockchain–The Untold Story' is the first ever book to be translated from English into Chinese by Artificial Engineering Bots.

Srinivas is the author of 'Corona Wars- Chronicles of a Corporate General", the world's first STEM fiction book written in April 2020, that delved in length about the Covid-19 pandemic and predicted accurately the origin and course of the Pandemic.

Srinivas is a founder of MMAPL, a cutting edge Blockchain consultancy & training company, through the e-Learning portal www.genuinitylabs.com .

www.ingramcontent.com/pod-product-compliance
Lightning Source LLC
Chambersburg PA
CBHW061358250726

48657CB00004B/1553